SENIOR STRENGTH
EXERCISES 60+

Over 150 Illustrated Home Exercises to Restore Energy, Build Strength, and Improve Balance and Flexibility

Written by William Patterson

DEDICATED

To my wife, Cheryl

Disclaimer Notice:

Please note that the information contained within this document is for educational and entertainment purposes only. All effort has been expended to present accurate, up-to-date, reliable, and complete information. No warranties of any kind are declared or implied. Readers acknowledge that the author is not engaged in the rendering of legal, financial, medical, or professional advice. The content within this book has been derived from various sources. Please consult a licensed professional before attempting any techniques outlined in this book.

By reading this document, the reader agrees that under no circumstances is the author responsible for any losses, direct or indirect, that are incurred as a result of the use of the information contained within this document, including, but not limited to, errors, omissions, or inaccuracies.

TABLE OF CONTENTS

ABDOMINALS AND OBLIQUES

UPPER BACK 220

LOWER BACK 239

Introduction

As a senior citizen, having a weekly exercise routine is one of the best things you can do for your health as we age. It can reduce the risk of heart disease, diabetes, osteoporosis, arthritis, and depression.

It also can boost your mood, improve your cognitive function, and help you sleep better at night. It can help prevent bone loss, enhance muscle strength and stamina, lessen the risk of falls, and improve balance. Bone-strengthening exercises can be aerobic, making your heart and lungs work harder than usual.

Everyday activities for bone health include running, walking, jumping rope, and strength exercises.

Yoga and tai chi are not as effective at strengthening bones but provide significant flexibility and balance benefits.

Another type of exercise is brisk walking, which can increase bone strength and exercise the heart. Brisk walking can also help prevent osteoporosis and other skeletal conditions with a healthy diet.

As we age, the internal scaffolding of our bones (including the vertebrae in our spine) loses calcium and other minerals. This results in a thin, brittle, and easily breakable bone density known as osteoporosis. The lubricating fluid inside your joints is also reduced, causing the cartilage to shrink, stiffen, and shorten. Ligaments are also weaker and more prone to wear, making it more challenging to move your joints freely. These changes are caused by a combination of age and lack of activity. But a daily workout program emphasizing weight-bearing and muscle-strengthening exercises can reverse these changes. Besides the right exercises, a healthy diet rich in vitamins and minerals can contribute to healthy bones.

Foods high in calcium and Vitamin D, such as dairy products, fish, and leafy green vegetables, can strengthen your bones and reduce the risk of fractures. And sun exposure may also boost the body's ability to absorb these nutrients.

As senior adults age, they often face emotional and social challenges that they may not have met. As a result, they are more susceptible to developing mental health disorders like depression and anxiety. Keeping up with exercise can help prevent and alleviate the symptoms of these mental health issues. Research has shown that regular physical activity can increase serotonin levels, which are nerve cells produced by the brain and spinal cord that help regulate attention, behavior, and body temperature and can ward off sadness and improve mood.

It also increases blood flow to the brain, which helps bring oxygen and other nutrients to its cells. This is important for memory and learning, as well as emotional health.

Exercising is an excellent way for seniors to stay mentally healthy. It gives seniors structure in their day, making them feel more energized and focused on their goals. Additionally, it can also help you combat feelings of loneliness.

Participating in a group fitness class can be a great way to meet new people and leave the house.

A recent study found that adults who participated in a program of aerobic exercise experienced a significant reduction in depressive symptoms. Another study reported that senior adults who exercised regularly had a lower risk of dementia, a common mental health problem among seniors.

If you are ready to begin with an unstoppable attitude, determination and are motivated to stick with it, you will be glad you did. Within the pages of this book, I will show you the illustrated exercises you will need to perform, starting with the neck and down throughout the entire body, covering all the major muscle groups.
Exercises using a small weight with the proper form are all you need to reach your fitness objective. With the human body being very adaptive, it will adapt to the slightest weight increases within your fitness routine, no matter who you are or your age.

Keep this one thing in mind, "Any Movement is Exercise," and any additional weight being used to exercise; you will see results. I have been involved in physical fitness for over 59 years. As I grew older, gym memberships were a part of my life. I Received my certified sports nutrition specialist certification in March 2011 and helped many on their journey to a healthier life through diet and fitness.

I received my personal certified fitness trainer certification in 2013 and helped clients of all ages develop strong and healthy bodies. To this day, I continue to strength train at least five days a week, sometimes more. Fitness strength training has been my life. My wife and I are a lot healthier and stronger because of it.

Now we would like to share our experiences with you. If you consistently follow the exercises in this book, you will be healthier and stronger, with more energy to live or continue living independently.

You will walk with that youthful strength and confidence, feeling strong with lots of energy at the start of each day.

You may have heard about endorphins, a feel-good chemical hormone your body releases during and after a workout. You will start feeling those endorphins after every workout. They will also help relieve pain, reduce stress, and improve your well-being. You'll start getting stronger, feeling like those younger years, thinking more clearly, and being able to pick up your grandkids and great-grands easily when they visit. Now is an excellent time to start your strength training exercises, do not wait. Please do it now. Enjoying added strength, energy, improved balance, and flexibility is just a decision away.

THE AGING PROCESS

Aging is the process by which we grow older. It occurs in humans and other animals, including plants, fungi, and bacteria. Some species are biologically immortal, such as simple animals and some perennials. However, they may show signs of aging at different rates. Aging is a general process that involves changes in the body's functions. This causes a decrease in adaptive responses to stress and can increase the risk for age-related diseases. People who are sixty years of age and older are elderly. Many diseases are related to aging but are not necessarily caused by aging. The aging process is associated with several biological, environmental, psychological, behavioral, and social changes. While many of these changes are benign (like graying hair), others may be harmful, such as an increased risk of heart disease, stroke, and dementia. Regardless of the causes, aging causes a decline in everyday activities and increases the likelihood of several chronic diseases.

The most informative actuarial function is the age-specific mortality rate, which Benjamin Gompertz discovered. His observation led to the development of the Gompertz function, which is derived by plotting death rates on a logarithmic scale. Interestingly, many diseases increase geometrically with the mortality rate, except for infectious diseases caused by a disturbed immune system. In summary, aging is a complex process, with several phases that overlap with each other. Aging is a process that involves loss of biological functions and decreased body ability to adapt to metabolic stress. However, aging can have positive effects. Those who age gracefully and with dignity will likely live long, healthy lives.

The global population is aging. Almost every nation is experiencing an increase in older adults. This process represents one of the most significant social transformations in the 21st century. It affects nearly every sector of society, including labor markets, family structures, and intergenerational ties. Therefore, it is essential to understand the impact of aging on society.

The Contributing Factors to the Aging Process

The pace of population aging is speeding up around the world. By 2050, two-thirds of the world's population over 60 years will live in low- and middle-income countries.

Aging is characterized by various molecular and cellular changes affecting health, mobility, and mental capacity. These include hearing loss, vision impairment, back pain, and arthritis.

Genetics

Our genes are the pieces of information that get passed down from one generation to the next. They tell our bodies how to make proteins and other essential body parts.

The field of genetics, which studies how traits and characteristics are determined and passed down, began in the mid-19th century with the work of a monk named Gregor Mendel. He noticed that pea plants that were crossbred in specific ways produced different colors of seeds.

Since then, researchers have discovered many other ways our genes influence our health and behavior. They are now searching for new ways to treat diseases and develop crops more resistant to pests or drought.

In addition to causing aging, many of our genetics affect how well we can heal ourselves from illnesses. For example, our bodies take longer to heal from a cut than when we were younger.

Environment

The environment that surrounds you is a significant contributing factor to the aging process. It includes everything from the soil and water to the animals and plants you live around.

Aging is a process of changes in the physical, psychological, and social aspects of an individual's life. It occurs due to environmental factors, including genetics, lifestyle, stress, and health.

The environment can also contribute to aging by providing opportunities for people to have healthy and active lives. For example, older adults can enjoy an exciting retirement community encouraging them to participate in new hobbies and activities.

Lifestyle

The lifestyle that you lead is an essential contributor to your aging process. Having a healthy diet, getting enough exercise, and cutting back on smoking and alcohol can help slow the rate at which you age.

Your social environment can also influence aging. It is essential to have stable relationships with family and friends, avoid stress and keep a good work-life balance.

These tips can help you age well and maintain a quality of life that allows you to enjoy your later years. You can also talk to your doctor about ways you can improve your health and reduce your risk of developing certain conditions that could affect your ability to live independently.

Aging is an important issue, as people worldwide live longer. It is expected that two-thirds of the world's population will be over sixty by 2050.

Stress

Stress is a common feature of everyday life and can be caused by many different situations. Examples include work-related pressures, financial worries, interpersonal relationships, and chronic illnesses.

The human body responds to stress by setting off a series of alarms, including releasing hormones that sharpen the senses, quicken the pulse, and deepen respiration. These are designed to help us defend against threatening situations.

However, prolonged stress can be a significant contributor to accelerated aging. This is because stress sets off a stress response that has long-lasting impacts on the brain, heart, and immune system.

In the case of the immune system, research suggests that stress may shorten telomeres, protective caps on the end of DNA chromosomes. This process cuts the life span of the chromosomes, accelerating the cellular aging process.

9 Effects of Senior Adult Exercise

Almost everyone knows the benefits of exercising, but older adults can reap even more from their workout routines. Regular physical activity can reduce the risk of several diseases and health conditions, including heart disease, diabetes, and osteoporosis.

Getting active can also improve senior citizens' ability to stay independent. This includes strengthening your bones, improving your balance, and making them more mobile.

1. <u>Strengthening of bones</u>

During regular senior citizen exercise, bones strengthen and develop. Stronger bones mean fewer fractures and better balance.

The loss of bone density in both men and women as we age is a significant health issue, particularly for post-menopausal women. However, strength training has been shown to help counter this loss and restore bone mass.

In addition to strengthening bones, this activity also increases muscle mass and improves overall mobility and flexibility. This helps seniors avoid falls, which can lead to severe injuries.

Physical activities that involve aerobics and strength training are critical to a healthy lifestyle for all age groups. Some aerobic exercises include walking, swimming, and riding a stationary bike.

2. **Increased stamina**

Exercise is a crucial part of healthy living. Not only does it reduce the risk of heart disease, diabetes, and osteoporosis, but it also helps increase your stamina and strengthen your bones.

As we age, we lose muscle mass and bone density and may find it difficult to perform simple tasks like walking up the stairs, going food shopping, or performing household chores. However, even a tiny amount of exercise can increase your stamina and help you perform daily activities.

Seniors can build their endurance through various activities, such as walking, gardening, swimming, or playing sports with friends. In addition to building strength, these activities are also great for improving mobility.

3. Decreased risk of heart disease

Senior citizen exercise is essential to maintaining a healthy heart and lungs. The Centers for Disease Control and Prevention (CDC) recommends that adults sixty-five and older get at least 150 minutes of moderate aerobic or cardiac exercise per week. This includes brisk walking, jogging, swimming, and cycling. Adding strength training to your routine is also a good idea, which can help maintain muscle mass and keep your weight in check.

A recent study found that seniors with a regular exercise routine had lower risks of heart problems than those who were sedentary. This was even true for people with disabilities and chronic conditions such as high blood pressure, high cholesterol levels, and diabetes.

Seniors can start exercising early and build up to a healthy level over time. A simple way to start is to walk 10,000 steps per day. This is equivalent to a quarter-mile walk, and it will improve your health and decrease your risk of illness.

4. Improved mental health

Stress is one of the most common challenges that seniors face in retirement, and exercise can be a great way to relieve stress. Regular exercise can also help improve the quality of sleep and prevent feelings of anxiety and depression.

A recent study showed that senior citizens who exercised regularly had better mental health than those who were sedentary. This is good news for those in charge of senior care, as physical activity can also help maintain senior citizens' independence and reduce their risk of falls.

Social interaction is another important factor in maintaining a senior citizen's mental health. Getting out and spending time with friends is essential to combat feelings of loneliness, and exercise can make this possible.

5. Decreased risk of diabetes

Aside from the benefits to general health and mental

well-being, exercise also helps seniors manage diabetes. It improves glycemic control, cardiovascular function, muscle strength, and functional capacity in diabetic older adults.

While exercising can involve various activities, experts recommend that senior citizens get at least 30 minutes of aerobic activity daily to improve blood sugar and insulin health. Ideally, they should include resistance and flexibility exercises as well.

However, if impact activities are too painful or not feasible, there are several ways to incorporate exercise into a busy lifestyle. One is to do yard work, which can burn up to 150 calories in 30-45 minutes.

Another way to incorporate exercise into a senior's routine is to do balance exercises regularly. These can be done while seated or standing. They can be a great way to reduce falls and improve balance in older adults with limited mobility.

6. Decreased risk of osteoporosis

Exercise can help your bones stay strong and reduce fall risk, which is significant for seniors. Put at least 30 minutes of moderate-intensity physical activity into your weekly schedule.

Strength activities, such as weightlifting, can increase bone density and decrease the risk of osteoporosis. They are also a great way to improve balance and increase muscle strength, an integral part of overall health.

Seniors should do stretching exercises at least two times each week. They can be done while watching TV or waiting for the kettle to boil. Stretching exercises can help your muscles warm up and prepare them for more strenuous workouts.

A recent study investigated the effect of exercise on bone mineral density (BMD) and fracture risk in postmenopausal women at high risk for osteoporosis. They found that women who regularly exercised had a lower risk of developing osteoporosis than those who did not exercise.

7. Decreased risk of depression

Exercise has several physical health benefits for seniors, including improving muscle strength and improving blood flow to the brain. It can also help prevent falls and bone fractures.

A new study has shown that moderately exercising senior citizens may help reduce depression. The researchers found that 30 minutes of exercise three times a week may help seniors deal with depression better than antidepressant drugs.

A recent study in Japan shows that older Japanese who exercised with others had a lower risk of developing depression five years later than those who did not exercise. The results of this study are similar to those found in other studies and could be an effective way for older adults to prevent the onset of mental health issues.

8. Decreased risk of dementia

Several studies have shown that physical activity can reduce the risk of dementia, especially Alzheimer's disease. Specifically, research has shown that aerobic exercise helps to slow shrinkage in the hippocampus, which is responsible for memory.

However, previous studies have been criticized for their limited sample sizes and lack of control for other health conditions, which may have led to biases.

One thousand seven hundred forty participants aged 65 years and above who did not have dementia were screened by the Cognitive Ability Screening.

Instrument (CASI) in the Adult Changes in Thought (ACT) study and followed biannually. Baseline measurements included exercise frequency, cognitive function, physical function, depression, health conditions, lifestyle characteristics, and other potential risk factors for dementia, such as the apolipoprotein E e4 allele.

9. Decreased risk of falls

It is crucial for senior citizens to realize that exercising is beneficial for their overall well-being and helps them stay active, healthy, and independent.

A recent study found that exercise can reduce the risk of falls by 23% in community-dwelling adults!

Exercise is a powerful way to decrease the risk of falling and increase your strength, stamina, and balance. Plus, it can be a fun social event, essential for senior citizens to keep them feeling a sense of purpose and prevent loneliness or depression.

Keeping fit and being active is also essential for your mental health, as it can decrease stress and anxiety and promote good sleep. Furthermore, it can help relieve the physical pain and stiffness that sometimes accompanies aging.

It is imperative for elderly individuals to get medical clearance from their doctor before starting an exercise program, as they may need to modify their workouts to prevent injury and other complications related to a preexisting condition.

The Centers for Disease Control and Prevention recommends a minimum of 150 minutes of moderate exercise per week to help maintain healthy body weight and improve muscle strength, stamina, and bone density.

A balanced diet is also essential for maintaining proper health, which can help reduce the likelihood of falls and other injuries as you age.

A recent Cochrane systematic review found that exercise can have a fall-prevention effect in community-dwelling older adults. However, this effect is more pronounced in those who engage in strength training. Therefore, further trials of fall-prevention exercise are needed to evaluate different types of physical activity and to examine how exercise is effective in other contexts.

What is the Cause of Muscle Stiffness?

Muscle stiffness can occur after a challenging workout, active trip, or vacation. It may also be a sign of an underlying health condition or side effect from medication.

Stiff muscles are a common symptom of many conditions, so it is essential to see your doctor when they interfere with your daily life. Your provider can use tests to identify the cause of your stiffness and prescribe a treatment plan.

Overuse injuries

Overuse injuries can develop when a muscle, tendon, ligament, or bone is repeatedly stressed and never gets a chance to heal. Stress fractures are a typical example of this. Overused muscles and tendons can also develop scar tissue in the area, which can cause nerve entrapment. Symptoms may include numbness, tingling, or pain. The best way to prevent overuse injuries is to understand how your body works and listen to it. Be sure to stretch before and after exercises and give your body time to recover between workouts. Stretching is as important as the exercise.

Muscle strains

A muscle strain is a common injury that can occur during exercise. They can be a one-time overstretching injury (acute injury) or an overuse injury that happens over time because of repetitive use.

Muscle strains are most common in muscles that rely on eccentric contraction. These fast-twitch muscles develop high-speed contractions, such as the hamstrings, gastrocnemius, quadriceps, and hip flexors.

Minor strains can usually be treated at home with rest, ice, and over-the-counter medicine. More severe strains may require surgical repair. Symptoms typically lessen within a few weeks but may take months to heal fully.

Muscle spasms

Several factors can cause muscle stiffness. However, it can also signify something more serious, especially if other symptoms are present.

Stiffness can also be a side effect of certain medications, like statins and anesthetics. If your doctor suspects an underlying condition is causing your muscle stiffness, they may run blood tests or take X-rays to identify the problem.

A person with muscle spasms can usually ease the discomfort by resting, applying gentle heat, or massage therapy. However, if the spasms become severe or last longer than a few days, seeking medical help is essential.

Infections

Infections occur when a microorganism (a pathogen) enters the body and causes harm. They can be bacteria, viruses, parasites, or fungi.

In some infections, the bacteria may overwhelm your immune system and cause severe symptoms. For example, pneumococci and staphylococci can infect the lungs, causing septicemia with high fever.

Some infectious diseases spread from person to person through coughing, sneezing, or contact with contaminated surfaces. Others are caused by bites from bugs or other animals that carry the bacteria. A well-rounded exercise program will strengthen the body and help fight infections and diseases.

Obesity

In addition to being a risk factor for heart disease and strokes, obesity also increases your risk of developing several severe health conditions, including chronic pain.

Obesity is generally caused by eating too many calories – particularly in fatty and sugary foods – and not burning off that excess energy through physical activity.

This extra weight puts a lot of stress on the joints in your body. As a result, it can cause joint stiffness and even lead to chronic joint problems such as osteoarthritis.

Arthritis

Arthritis affects the body's joints, which are where bones meet. These joints contain cartilage, a smooth substance that protects and cushions the ends of bones.

When arthritis occurs, this cartilage breaks down, and the bone ends rub together. This can happen for many reasons, including autoimmune diseases or injury.

Symptoms include pain, stiffness, and decreased joint movement. They may also be accompanied by swelling, redness, and tenderness.

Inflammation

Inflammation is your body's natural way of fighting infection and repairing tissue damage. It increases blood flow and immune cells to a specific area, where they identify and attack germs, toxins, or other intruders.

However, inflammation can also be problematic when it goes too far and causes chronic disease. It can increase your risk of heart disease, cancer, Alzheimer's, and other conditions.

Stiffness caused by an underlying health condition is often treated with over-the-counter pain relievers and stronger medications if needed. It is important to tell your doctor about all your symptoms, including stiffness, to get an accurate diagnosis.

7 Tips to Maximize Your Workouts and Minimize Injuries

Exercise is a critical part of healthy aging, and it helps older adults improve strength and reduce the risk of falls. But if you do not follow certain safety precautions, even the most moderate workout can cause injury.

The best way to stay safe is by exercising with proper technique and staying hydrated. These seven tips will help you minimize the risk of an injury and ensure your workouts are a positive experience!

1. <u>Warm Up</u>

A warm-up is essential to a workout and should be performed before physical activity. It helps the body prepare for more intense work and decreases the chance of injury.

An effective warm-up increases your heart rate and blood flow, allowing additional oxygen to enter your muscles. It also helps to stretch your muscles and increase flexibility.

Generally, an effective warm-up takes about 10 to 15 minutes, says Sabrena Jo, director of science and research content at the American Council on Exercise. However, seniors with arthritis or a heart condition may need more time to warm up properly.

The best warm-up type includes gentle cardiovascular exercise and dynamic stretching, including movements that mimic those you will do during your workout. Light calisthenics like squats and push-ups are often used to warm up the large muscle groups, while low-weight strength training exercises can be included in the warm-up to challenge your smaller muscle groups.

A good warm-up is also crucial because it can improve your mental health and reduce stress. Studies show that warming up helps elevate your core temperature, which makes it easier to stretch your muscles and decreases stiffness.

2. **Wear the Right Shoes**

Investing in the right shoes for seniors is one of the best things that you can do to help reduce your risk of falling. The right shoes can also make you feel more comfortable, increasing your chances of staying healthy and active for longer.

When looking for a shoe, it is essential to consider your foot shape and size. This will ensure that the shoes are not too tight or too loose.

A shoe that does not fit properly can restrict the foot and impair balance and walking. It is essential for seniors with poor balance and coordination.

In addition to the correct foot shape, it is also essential that the shoes have a low heel and slip-resistant sole. This will reduce the chance of slipping and falling, especially in wet weather.

When shopping for the right pair of shoes, it is essential to take a little time and try on a few different styles and brands. Ideally, try them on both feet to see how they feel and walk around for a while to get a feel for how they fit.

3. Start Slowly

Starting too quickly is one of the biggest reasons seniors get injured during exercise. Instead, increase your workouts slowly over time. Start with 5 minutes of slow walking several times daily, then add a few more each week. Once you are comfortable, try a more extended exercise session, such as jogging, biking, or swimming for 30 minutes most days of the week.

Getting in shape can help older adults live longer, healthier lives. It can also prevent falls and broken bones. In addition, exercise can boost your energy levels and help you sleep better at night.

4. Stay Hydrated

Whether you are a seasoned athlete or enjoy exercising for fun, it is essential to stay hydrated during any workout. Dehydration can lead to muscle cramps, dizziness, and other severe symptoms. A great way to stay hydrated is by drinking water before, during, and after any exercise or activity. You can also drink beverages like low-sugar sports drinks and protein shakes designed for seniors.

Another good way to stay hydrated during a workout is by eating foods high in water content. Vegetables and fruits like cucumbers, tomatoes, watermelon, and spinach contain a lot of water, so it is essential to include these in your diet daily. If you are unsure how much water you should drink daily, talk to your doctor or other health care professional. Generally, people should aim to drink about 15 cups of water daily. If you have difficulty remembering to drink enough water, set up a routine and make it part of your daily habits. Try to drink a glass of water first thing in the morning, before you shower, and with each meal.

5. **Cool Down**

After a workout, it is essential to cool down properly. Doing so can help prevent injury and ensure your body is ready for the next workout.

Warming up and cooling down can be difficult for seniors, especially when they are new to exercise. However, it is essential to remember that the two can be performed together.

While a warmup prepares your body for the intense exercise you will be doing, a cool-down helps to slow down your heart rate and blood pressure so that you do not become dizzy or faint during a workout.

It also helps to decrease the risk of rotator cuff injuries. You can do this by reducing the amount of weight you are using during your workout or by choosing an activity that does not put as much stress on your shoulders and rotator cuffs.

An excellent cool-down routine should include gentle jogging or walking to allow your heart rate to slow down and your blood to return to normal. You should also stretch to decrease muscle tightness and restore the length of your muscles.

6. Take a Break

Taking a break during your workout can give your muscles, mind, and body a chance to recover from the stress of your workout. It can also allow you to switch to a different activity.

If you have trouble concentrating during your workout, step away from the machine or the weights and do some easy-to-do exercises like walking or stretching. This can help you feel energized and refreshed when you return to your work.

Taking a break when you need it is essential, not when you think you should! The right amount of rest will prevent you from overreaching and overtraining, which can lead to aches and pains in the body. Another way to get a break is by going outside. Being around nature can improve your mood, help you relax, and even help you find solutions to a problem.

7. **See Your Doctor**

If you are a senior, seeing your doctor before you start an exercise routine is essential. This is especially true if you have health conditions like heart disease or diabetes, which may limit your ability to work out safely.

A healthy lifestyle is essential to age well, and getting regular physical activity is one of the best ways for seniors to improve their health. It also helps you maintain independence and fight off diseases, such as heart disease or diabetes.

While most workout injuries will heal independently,

seeing your doctor if you experience pain or other symptoms when exercising is still a good idea. Your doctor can advise you on the best types of exercise and how to do them safely.

Taking a break from exercising is a good idea if you get injured until you're fully healed. You might also need to consult your doctor if you continue to feel pain or have difficulty performing activities you previously enjoyed. For example, if your knees hurt when you run, try a different exercise or change the intensity.

6 Exercises to Improve Your Balance

Whether you are just starting a healthy lifestyle or looking to enhance your current routine, improving your balance is a great way to keep yourself safer. You can do a few simple exercises at home to improve your balance and help prevent falls. These exercises are manageable but require patience and consistency as you progress.

1. **Mini Squats**

Mini squats are one of the best exercises for boosting your balance. They also help you build strength, reducing your risk of injury and helping you improve your posture.

Mini squats are a popular exercise that targets the quads, glutes, and hamstrings. Strong legs are crucial to reducing the risk of falls and injury, which can be particularly dangerous for older adults.

A typical squat involves standing about shoulder-width apart and keeping your feet parallel. If you have hip issues, you may prefer a slightly wider stance. Holding the back of a stable chair or any stable object, lower your body as far as possible, then back up again. A complete illustration is given in the quadriceps section of this book.

Squats are one of the best balance exercises for seniors, but you should always talk to your doctor before trying a new exercise. They can tell you if it is safe for you and give you tips on safely performing the movement.

2. Heel raises

Heel raises strengthen your calf muscles, which help with walking, jumping, and climbing steps. They also make your ankles more stable and less likely to get injured.

One of the most basic balance exercises for seniors, heel raises, is easy to do. They require just a tiny amount of support, such as a wall, table, or chair.

Start by standing in front of a sturdy chair with your feet hip-width apart. Slowly lift your right foot straight back without bending your knee or pointing your toes, holding this position for a few seconds, then slowly lower it to the floor.

Repeat this exercise ten times per leg to improve your balance. If you need help, place your hands on a countertop or hold onto the back of a stable chair.

Heel raises can be difficult for some people, but they do not need to be painful. If you notice any pain or discomfort during exercise, stop and rest until it disappears.

Heel raises are also an effective exercise for reducing

pain in the Achilles tendon, which runs from your heel to your knee. They can be particularly helpful for those who have Achilles tendinitis.

3. Leaning forward

Balance is an important skill to maintain and build on as we age. It is essential for walking and navigating stairs and can help prevent falls in seniors.

As you age, your muscles may weaken, and your joints lose flexibility. These changes can lead to a loss of balance, so performing exercises that strengthen the core and improve coordination is vital.

Leaning forward is a great exercise to work on balance. It can also help relieve pain in the back if you have arthritis.

To do this exercise, stand with your feet shoulder-width apart and hold on to a sturdy chair. This is an excellent first step to regaining your balance and a fun way to involve the whole family!

The key to leaning forward is to bend your hips. This will give you the added support you need to keep your body stable as you bend forward.

This senior balance exercise is also a great way to

strengthen your legs and improve your coordination. To do this, stand with your feet shoulder-width apart and lift your left leg out to the side while slowly pushing off with your right foot. Repeat with the other leg and stay in this position for 10 seconds.

Leaning forward is common among athletes trying to accelerate quickly and stay balanced. It is also helpful in sports like golf, where the player needs to be able to lean forward and still be always upright.

4. Marching

Marching is a common and effective balance exercise for seniors. It can also improve mobility and strengthen lower limb muscles, reducing the risk of falls.

It is also a great core exercise that can be done standing up, which is vital for improving strength and balance. However, being safe when performing these exercises is essential: you should never do these without a wall or other support.

It would be best if you started with easy balance exercises before progressing to more challenging ones. Talk to your doctor about which balance exercises are right for you.

Then, practice these bodyweight exercises as often as possible. They will help you feel more confident as you go about your day.

Once you are comfortable with the routine, perform it with more weight or resistance. You may want to use a small kettlebell or another weighted object for added challenges.

In addition to improving your balance, these exercises are also great for strengthening your neck muscles.

Just be sure to keep your head still when you're doing them so you don't strain your neck or back.

5. **Side leg raises**

Side leg raises are a great exercise to help seniors improve their balance. They are a bodyweight exercise that strengthens the Gluteus Medius muscle, which helps you maintain your balance when standing or walking.

These exercises can be performed from a variety of positions, so they are easy to do at home or in the gym. They are also great for improving core strength. The most important thing to keep in mind when doing a side-leg raise is to avoid locking your knees. Locking your knees can lead to pain and injury.

Performing this exercise correctly can strengthen your hip abductor muscles, which are the primary muscle groups that control hip movement.

This exercise can be made more challenging by adding small weights. Start with two pounds and increase as your strength increases.

Another option is to add resistance bands around your thighs. These make the exercise harder, but they also decrease the torque on your hip and knee.

To perform this exercise, lie on your side and lift one leg about six inches off the floor, then lower it back down. Repeat this a few times.

This is a great exercise to target the often-overlooked gluteal muscles. It can be added to your workout routine as a warm-up or end-of-workout stretch.

6. Walking

Walking is a simple and effective balance exercise for seniors. It also promotes overall health and improves cognitive functioning in seniors.

Research has shown that regular walking helps

seniors manage chronic diseases like heart disease, diabetes, and stroke. In addition, it lowers their risk of falling and injury by increasing muscle strength.

The CDC recommends that adults walk at least 30 minutes per day. It is easy, affordable, and requires no special equipment or training (Morris & Hardman, 1997).

If you are not an avid walker, try to get inspired to walk more by remembering the health benefits of it. Find creative ways to get up and move, such as going for a walk in a park or walking in the community. Studies have found that positive-framed messages are more effective at promoting walking than negative-framed messages in older adults. However, the effect is not as strong in young adults.

Dynamic Stretches and Their Benefits

Dynamic stretches will help reduce injury and increase strength and flexibility, which will help you move better during your workout. In addition, dynamic stretches can help you become more aware of your body. They mimic the movements you will be performing during your workout and improve body awareness. Start with simple, slow movements and work up to more difficult ones as you get more flexible. Dynamic stretches can improve flexibility and reduce the risk of injury during a run. They can also help you become more robust; however, it is essential to do them within the range of motion you are currently comfortable with. The longer you do them, the more your range of motion will improve.

There are two types of stretches: static stretches and dynamic stretches. While static stretches require you to hold the muscles in one position for 15 to 30 seconds, dynamic stretches use active movements to prepare your muscles for intense activity. They can also serve as warm-up exercises before exercise and improve your workouts. An example of a dynamic stretch is the knee-to-chest exercise. You performed by bringing your knee toward your chest before lowering your foot toward the ground. This is done by alternating each leg while walking or standing stationary. Dynamic stretches involve movement, improving your range of motion. Because they involve movement, dynamic stretches increase blood flow in your muscles and help you avoid injury. Dynamic stretches are significant for runners because they target essential muscles like your arms, shoulders, and core. One study showed that runners who practiced Dynamic stretches before a run improved their endurance. Performing a dynamic stretch is an effective way to improve your overall health. Stretching can help increase your circulation, which delivers oxygen and nutrients throughout the body. It can also help alleviate muscle tightness, soreness, and stiffness. Plus, it can help you stay in tip-top shape and improve your posture.

Static Stretches and Their Benefits

Among the many benefits of static stretches is the ability to alleviate arthritis and relieve pain. These stretches can also help improve mobility and flexibility and are usually performed at the end of your workout. Performing static stretches can be an effective way to relax your muscles and increase your flexibility. This is especially true after that workout.

Stretching daily is a great way to improve your overall health. It is also an effective way to increase your range of motion and reduce muscle pain. A good stretching routine can help you live a longer, healthier life. A static stretching routine should be straightforward. Choosing a few challenging static stretches to work on is a good idea. It would be best to select stretches that prioritize certain muscle groups. It is important to remember to breathe deeply while stretching. This can be a great way to boost your circulation and deliver more oxygen to your muscles.

Stretching to Relieve Arthritis

Whether you have arthritis or someone who wants to relieve arthritis pain, static stretching is a great way to reduce joint pain and improve joint function. It does not matter where your irritation may be. A good stretch regularly will help improve your movement. You may also choose to do static stretches randomly during the day. You can do these stretches in bed, sitting in a chair, or standing. Talking with your doctor about your specific symptoms and medical condition is essential before starting any exercise routine.

Stretches to Prevent Injuries

Performing static stretches to prevent injuries for seniors can help improve their health and quality of life. They can improve mobility, alleviate muscle pain, and even improve brain function. Performing a few simple stretches is easy to do and can be incorporated into any daily routine. Performing static stretches can also help maintain full-body mobility. Static stretching improves muscle flexibility, which improves coordination and balance. Performing stretches can also increase circulation and decrease aches and pains. Having flexibility in your body is an essential part of good health. It improves daily functioning and reduces the risk of injury. Whether you are a senior or a young adult, it is essential to maintain your flexibility. Tight muscles can cause pain and strain and limit your range of motion.

Stretching is an excellent way to release this tension. It also helps to improve your posture. It allows your muscles to function correctly and supply nutrients to your body. It is a great way to improve your health, especially if you are older. Having flexibility in your body will also help reduce your risk of falling. It can also improve your balance and help you to climb stairs. When seniors perform static stretches, they can increase their flexibility and strength. They can also help to improve their balance. Stretches can be performed at home, with a caregiver, or in a group setting.

The best stretches for seniors focus on flexibility, balance, and posture. An excellent flexibility stretch is the standing hamstring stretch, which stretches the neck, back, glutes, hamstrings, and calves. This stretch is illustrated in this book's legs (hamstrings) section. These stretches can help improve blood circulation and increase the supply of oxygen and nutrients to the body. They also can reduce the risk of injury and help to prevent pain.

Pre-Workout Warm-up

The purpose of a warm-up is to prepare you mentally and physically for the demands of the exercises you will be performing. A warm-up is a gradual way to prepare your body for exercise. There is nothing wrong with a complete body warm-up you will get from riding a recumbent bike or light jogging. This will increase your heart rate and warm your body for the exercise movements to come. After this initial warm-up, I recommend warming the muscles you exercise just before the actual strength-building exercise.   This is done by dynamically stretching the muscle area being worked on. For example, if you are performing an arm exercise, your warm-up should involve the arm muscles you are preparing to exercise. If the exercise involves small dumbbells or kettlebells or any other type of small weight, go through one set of the workout without weights before performing the normal set with weights. This will flush blood to that specific area, warming the muscle and making it more flexible. After warming up the muscles in this way, begin your workout with the desired weight.

This warm-up technique should be followed for each weighted exercise listed in this book. As your strength increases for each exercise, begin using a heavier weight. Your warm-up may consist of a lighter weight as a warm-up set before the normal weight.   In other words, a very light version of the actual exercise. This will ensure that the muscle being exercised is directly warmed up. This is a technique to use once your strength level improves and you are using heavier weights. If you are there already, this technique is used most often to reduce muscle injury.

Doing a proper stretch can be difficult for seniors, but this is the way to improve your flexibility and improve your overall health. Performing a proper stretch can help you feel younger and improve your posture. A good stretch will also help you get your heart rate up, improve your circulation, and strengthen your muscles. These can all contribute to an overall healthier you. You can still stretch most of your major muscle groups from a seated position if you have limited mobility. To ensure that you are doing it properly, follow the guidelines in this book for the proper technique. You should also consult with your doctor or physical therapist before starting any exercise routine to ensure it is the right thing for your fitness level.

The best way to stretch your muscles is to focus on the major muscle groups. Stretching can also help reduce muscle stiffness, making daily tasks much more manageable. Stretching is an essential fitness component, but most people skip the stretch before they start their workout. Performing a few minutes of stretching before you start your workout can boost your performance and reduce your risk of injury. Performing a stretch regularly can also help improve your posture. By strengthening your muscles, you can maintain a good posture for years.

Post-Workout Cool-Down

A post-workout cool-down routine is a great way to ensure your body has time to heal and recover from a challenging workout. This is important because your heart rate may be slightly elevated for a few hours following a workout. It is essential to take a moment to slow down your pace and breathe deeply to help your heart recover, so a cool down will help return your heart rate to a more normal level.

Cooling down is important because it helps reduce muscle soreness and prevent injury. It also helps your body regain homeostasis, which is its natural state after a workout. It will help to reduce the amount of lactate in the blood, which is an organic acid that causes muscle burn.

Static stretching is an effective way to relax your muscles to cool down. It can also help to increase blood flow to muscles, which can help them to heal and recover faster, increasing flexibility, which reduces the risk of injury.

It will help to alleviate muscle pain, which can occur

between 24 and 48 hours after a workout. Cooling down is also a great way to relax, which will help you get the most out of your workout. Taking a long meditative static stretch will help to relax your mind.

When you are trying to get a workout in, it is easy to try and cut corners and skip the cool down. I recommend ensuring you factor it in as part of your workout routine. The benefits far outweigh the disadvantages, especially if you are short of time.

NECK

The Benefits of Strengthening the Neck

The primary function of the cervical spine is to support the head and neck. It contains seven vertebrae, numbered from C1 to C7. The cervical spine has the most extensive range of motion of any vertebra in the human body. The first cervical vertebra, the atlas, is ring-shaped and connects directly to the skull. This allows for the head to nod. The second cervical vertebra is peg-shaped and has a projection called the odontoid. Both structures provide for side-to-side motion of the head and neck. The muscles of the neck perform several different functions. They are grouped into three major groups: anterior, lateral, and posterior. These groups are further subdivided according to function and depth. The neck muscles can also be grouped depending on the direction of their fibers. In addition to the three main muscle groups, some smaller muscles function differently. The neck muscles work together to stabilize the head and help with movements. They also help with swallowing and support the hyoid bone (The hyoid bone is in the front of the neck, just below the lower jaw, carrying the weight of the tongue and playing a vital role in speech and swallowing). In addition, these muscles are responsible for generating facial expressions.

The sternocleidomastoid is the primary muscle in the anterior(front) part of the neck. The lateral neck muscles include rectus capitis anterior and rectus capitis lateralis, two muscles that control head movements from the base of your skull. Longus capitis and longus coli are two muscles that help twist your head from side to side and twist and tilt your cervical spine. The posterior (Rear) neck muscles are responsible for the neck extension. Exercises that focus on the neck are not only beneficial for seniors, but they can benefit any age group. Another critical benefit of strengthening your neck muscles is that it improves your posture and reduces your risk of injury.

As we age, the spine becomes more brittle, making neck exercises essential to a senior's wellness routine. In addition to improving posture, exercises for the neck can also help you increase your mobility while keeping the muscles in the neck strong. In addition, even simple household activities like washing the dishes or picking up the mail can help tone up the neck muscles. These muscles help support the head and prevent pain. While many people do not realize it, moving your head up and down and side to side in your daily routine will help keep your neck and shoulders in shape. Do not forget that any movement is exercise. A tight neck can lead to painful symptoms such as arthritis or a nagging headache. However, a relaxed neck improves blood flow to the head, enhancing brain function. Remember, talking with your doctor about your specific symptoms and medical condition before starting any new exercise program is essential.

Illustrated Neck Strengthening Exercises

Seated

Muscle groups activated by the seated neck extension:

◆ Splenius cervicis and capitis

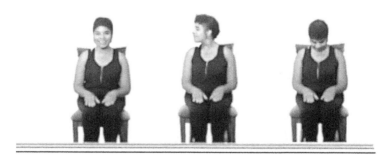

Seated Neck Extension:

Perform Seated, Standing or Lying Down:

To Begin:

1. Sit with your legs straight, keeping your

shoulders relaxed.

2. Hold your head up in neutral and look behind your right shoulder.

3. Hold this position for approximately 20 seconds and then rest for 1-minute.

4. Lower your head towards your chest and hold for 20 seconds.

5. Complete three sets of 5 to 10 reps, switching sides, and increase your sets or reps when your strength permits. Wait at least 1-minute in-between sets.

Muscle groups activated by the neck protraction stretch:

- Semispinalis cervicis
- Longissimus cervicis
- Spinalis cervicis
- Splenius cervicis

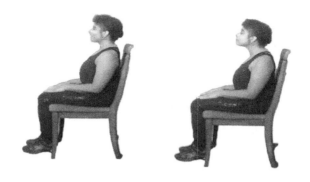

Seated Neck Protraction Stretch:

Perform Seated, Standing or Lying Down:

To Begin:

1. Sit upright comfortably in a good spinal position.
2. Gently move your head forward, pointing your chin away.
3. When your chin moves forward, the lower neck flexes.
4. Complete three sets of 5 to 10 reps, increase your reps, sets or both or sets when your strength increases. Wait at least 1-minute in-between sets.

Muscle groups activated by the neck flexion stretch:

- ◆ Sternocleidomastoid
- ◆ Anterior scalene
- ◆ Longus capitis and colli

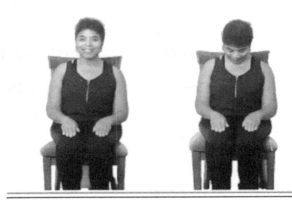

Seated Neck Flexion Stretch:

Perform Seated, Standing or Lying Down:

To Begin:

1. Bring the head forward so the chin touches the chest and the face looks downwards towards the floor.
2. Maintain the position briefly and slowly bring the head to the neutral position.
3. Neck flexion is assisted by the contraction of

neck muscles in front of the neck.

4 .   Neck flexion simultaneously stretches the back of the cervical spine muscle.

5 .   Complete three sets of 5 to 10 reps, increase your reps, sets or both when your strength increases. Wait at least 1-minute in-between sets.

Muscle groups activated by the seated lateral neck stretch:

◆   Levator Scapulae
◆   Upper Back (trapezius and rhomboids)

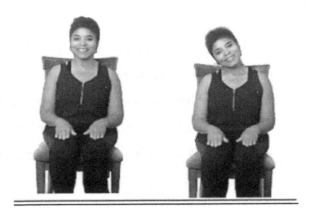

Seated Lateral Neck Stretch:

Perform Seated, Standing or Lying Down:

To Begin:

1. Sit upright comfortably in a good spinal position, shoulder back and relaxed.
2. Look forward while keeping your head up.
3. Slowly move your ear towards your right shoulder, do not lift your shoulder to your ear.
4. The head should be tilted for at least five seconds. Repeat on the left side.
5. Complete at least three sets of 5 to 10 reps, increase your reps, sets or both when your strength increases. Wait at least 1-minute in-between sets.

74

Standing

Muscle groups activated by the standing neck stretches:

◆ Sternocleidomastoid muscle

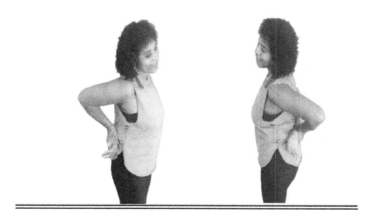

Standing Neck Stretches:

Perform Standing or Seated:

To Begin:

1. Stand straight with your feet hip-width apart, with your hands behind your back, grab your left wrist with your right hand, and bring it toward your right hip.

2. Bend your torso to the right and gently drop your right ear toward your right shoulder.

3. Complete three sets of 10 to 15 reps alternating to each side, increasing when your strength permits. Wait at least 1-minute in-between sets.

Muscle groups activated by the neck rolls:

◆ Cervical spine
◆ Neck muscles

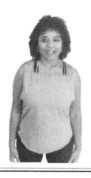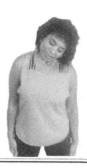

Neck Rolls:

Perform Standing or Seated:

To Begin:

1. Begin with your head straight and looking forward.
2. Tilt your head to the left and start rolling it back.
3. Keep rolling your head to the left and then down.
4. Bring your head up to the starting position and repeat in the opposite direction.
5. Complete three sets of 5 to 10 reps, increase your reps, sets or both when your strength increases. Wait at least 1-minute in-between sets.

Maintain your shoulders relaxed and keep the movements big, slow, and fluid. Breathe deeply and stretch the neck gently without letting it fall too far backward. You can start with a semicircular motion if your neck is too weak or uncomfortable. Drop the chin toward the chest and roll your head to the left, roll it back to the front and around to the right shoulder.

Muscle groups activated by the lateral neck stretch:

- Rectus Capitis, Anterior and Lateralis
- Longus Capitis

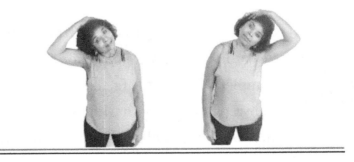

Lateral Neck Stretch:

Perform Standing or Seated:

To Begin:

1. Place your right hand on top of your head and gently tilt your head to the right.
2. Apply some pressure on your head with your hand to increase the stretch.
3. Hold this position for 10 - 15 seconds and repeat on the other side.
4. Complete three sets holding 10 to 15 seconds, increase your reps, sets or both when your strength increases. Wait at least 1-minute in-between sets.

Muscle groups activated by the nose circles:

◆ Upper Back (trapezius and rhomboids)

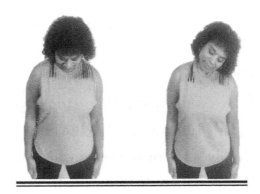

Nose Circles:

Perform Standing, Seated or Lying Down:

To Begin:

1. Stand with chin toward chest, then gently turn left ear toward left shoulder.

2. Focus gaze on the tip of your nose, draw ten tiny circles with the nose in one direction, and then do ten in the opposite direction.

3. Do not make big circles with your nose lifting toward the ceiling.

4. Keep movements small and go slowly.

5. When finished, return your head to the center and repeat on the other side.

6. Complete three circles on each side, doing ten in each direction. Increase your rep, sets or both

when your strength increases. Wait at least 1-minute in-between sets.

Lying Down

Muscle groups activated by the chin nod:

◆ Longus Colli and Capitis

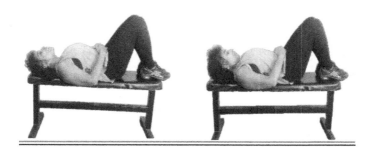

Chin Nodding:

Perform Lying Down, Seated or Standing:

To Begin:

1. Gently and slowly nod as if to say 'yes.'
2. Feel the muscles at the front of your neck.
3. Stop nodding just before you feel the front muscles hardening.
4. Hold the nod position for five seconds and then

relax.

5 . Gently move your head back to the usual start position.

6 . Complete three sets of ten each, increase your reps, sets or both, sets or both when your strength increases. Wait at least 1-minute in-between sets.

Muscle groups activated by the head rotation stretch.

◆   Sternocleidomastoid muscle
◆   Splenius Capitis
◆   Splenius Cervicis

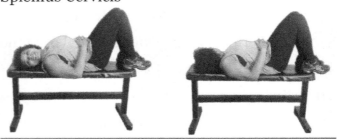

Head Rotation Stretch:

Perform Lying Down, Seated or Standing:

To Begin:

1. Gently turn your head from one side to the other.
2. Progressively aim to turn your head far enough to align your chin with your shoulder. And you can see the wall in line with your shoulder.
3. Complete three sets of 5 to 10 reps, increase your reps, sets or both when your strength increases. Wait at least 1-minute in-between sets.

Muscle groups activated by the hanging neck:

- Sternocleidomastoid
- Anterior scalene
- Longus Capitis
- Longus Colli

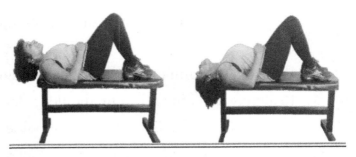

Hanging Neck Exercise:

Perform Lying Down, Seated or Standing:

To Begin:

1. Lie on a bench or bed with your shoulders near the edge.
2. Gently hang your head back over the edge of the bench or bed.
3. Hold this position for up to 1-minute.
4. Gently move your head back onto the bed or bench and relax in this position.
5. Complete three sets of 5 to 10 reps, increase your reps, sets or both when your strength increases. Wait at least 1-minute in-between sets.

SHOULDERS

The Benefits of Strengthening the Shoulders

The shoulder is an important joint that allows a person to move his or her arm in a wide range of motions. It must be stable and mobile enough to perform various arm functions, including lifting, pushing, and pulling. Senior citizens can exercise their shoulders by performing the exercises listed below. These exercises help to increase the range of motion in the shoulders and promote the ability to lift and pull. Exercising your shoulders can enhance your balance and reduce the risk of falling. As a result, you can walk with more confidence. If you continue these exercises regularly, your overall confidence will improve, and you will be more able to perform the activities you love without difficulty. Exercise of the shoulders can help you maintain your balance. Lack of balance can result in serious falls, which can have devastating consequences. You should have your bone density tested to ensure you're not at risk of falling. You risk falling if your bone density is low; weight-bearing exercises will help correct this problem. As we age, we naturally lose muscle mass. This can leave us weaker and more prone to injury. Weight-bearing exercises help to make your bones stronger and denser, and the muscles you develop with this type of exercise provide a significant amount of support to your bones. Along with better bones, weight-bearing exercises also help protect your joints by increasing your body's coordination, balance, and flexibility. A shoulder strength exercise program should be performed as a lifelong maintenance routine. Doing shoulder exercises two to three times a week will help maintain your strength and range of motion.

_____

Illustrated Shoulder Strengthening Exercises

Seated

Muscle groups activated by the shoulder shrug:

◆ Shoulders (anterior, medial, posterior deltoids)
◆ Upper Back (trapezius and rhomboids)

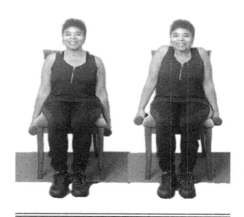

Seated Shoulder Shrug:

Perform Seated or Standing:

To Begin:

1. Sit comfortably in a good spinal position, holding a dumbbell or any weighted object in each hand. Shoulders back and Relaxed, looking straight ahead. Slowly raise both shoulders.
2. Hold for 5 seconds, then return to the starting position.
3. It should be done frequently during the day.
4. Complete three sets of 5 to 10 reps, increase your weight when your strength increases. Wait at least 1-minute in-between sets.

Note: Use light dumbbells of 1 to 2 pounds in the beginning; you can also use any weighted object, such as canned food items or any small, weighted items.

Muscle group activated by the seated dumbbell front raises:

- Shoulder (anterior deltoids, posterior deltoids)
- Upper Back (trapezius and rhomboids)
- Chest (pectoralis major)
- Arms (biceps)

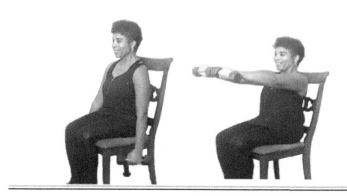

Seated Dumbbell Front Raises:

Perform Seated or Standing

To Begin:

1. Sit with a dumbbell in each hand at your side. With your back straight and your core activated.
2. With the elbows slightly bent or extended, raise the dumbbells in front of you, with your palms facing down, until your hands are just above shoulder height.
3. Lower the dumbbells back down and repeat.
4. Complete three sets of 5 to 10 reps, increase your weight when your strength increases. Wait at least 1-minute in-between sets.

Note: Use light dumbbells of 1 to 2 pounds in the beginning. You can also use any weighted object, such as canned food or small, weighted items.

Muscle groups activated by the seated dumbbell shoulder press:

- ◆ Shoulders (anterior, medial, posterior deltoids)
- ◆ Arms (triceps)
- ◆ Upper Back (trapezius and rhomboids)
- ◆ Chest (pectoralis major and minor)

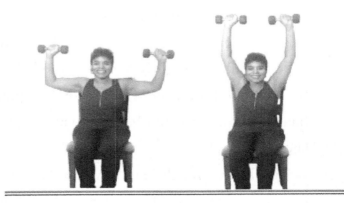

Seated Dumbbell Shoulder Press:

Perform Seated or Standing:

To Begin:

1. Sit with your legs shoulder-width apart and hold a dumbbell in each hand.
2. With your palms facing forward and your elbows under your wrists, position the dumbbells at your shoulders, with your upper arm parallel to the floor.
3. Push the dumbbells up without fully locking out your elbows.
4. Lower the dumbbells back down to your shoulders and repeat the movement until the set is complete.
5. Complete three sets of 5 to 10 reps; increase your weight when your strength increases. Wait at least 1-minute in-between sets.

Note: Use light dumbbells of 1 to 2 pounds in the beginning; you can also use any weighted object, such as canned food items or any small, weighted items.

Muscle groups activated by the seated alternating dumbbell shoulder press:

◆ Shoulders (anterior deltoids)
◆ Arms (triceps)
◆ Upper Back (trapezius and rhomboids)
◆ Chest (pectoralis major and minor)

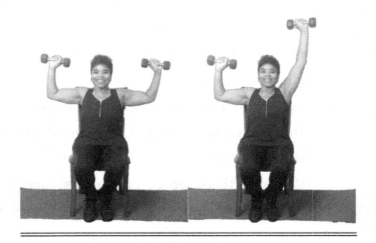

Seated Alternating Dumbbell Shoulder Press:

Perform Seated or Standing:

To Begin:

1. Sit with your feet hip-width apart.

2. Hold a dumbbell in each hand just above shoulder height with your palms facing forward

and arms bent.

3. Press one dumbbell over your head without moving the other. Slowly return to the start.

4. Press the other dumbbell over your head without moving the other dumbbell.

5. Return to the starting position.

6. Complete three sets of 5 to 10 reps, depending on your strength level.

7. Increase your weight when your strength level permits. Wait at least 1-minute in-between sets.

Note: Use light dumbbells of 1 to 2 pounds in the beginning; you can also use any weighted object, such as canned food items or any small, weighted items.

_____

Standing

Muscle groups activated by the standing side shoulder raise:

◆   Shoulders (medial deltoid)

◆ Arms (triceps)

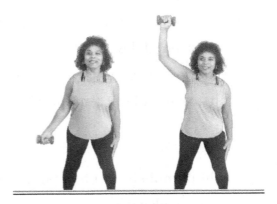

Standing Side Shoulder Raises:
Perform Standing or Seated

To Begin:

1. Begin with your right arm at your side, elbow straight, holding a dumbbell with your palms forward.

2. Raise your right arm outward to the side, with your elbows slightly bent and overhead.

3. Return to the starting position and repeat with

94

your left arm.

4. Complete three sets of 5 to 10 reps.

5. Increase your weight when your strength permits. Wait at least 1-minute in-between sets.

Note: Use light dumbbells of 1 to 2 pounds in the beginning; you can also use any weighted object, such as canned food items or any small, weighted items.

_____

Muscle groups activated by the standing shoulder roll:

- ◆ Shoulders (anterior and posterior deltoid)
- ◆ Upper Back (trapezius and rhomboids)
- ◆ Chest (pectoralis major and minor)

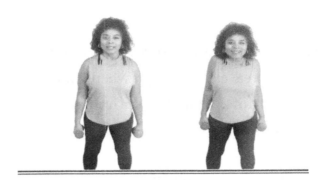

Standing Shoulder Roll:

Perform Standing, Seated or Lying Down:

To Begin:

1. Stand with your arms down at your sides, holding a dumbbell in each hand, with your palms facing each other.
2. Roll your shoulders backward in a circular motion, completing five rotations.
3. Then complete five rotations forward.
4. Repeat this sequence in three sets of 5-10 reps; increase your weight when your strength increases. Wait at least 1-minute in-between sets.

Note: Use light dumbbells of 1 to 2 pounds in the beginning; you can also use any weighted object, such as canned food items or any small, weighted items.

Muscle groups activated by the elbow side extensions:

◆ Shoulders (anterior deltoids, rear deltoid)
◆ Upper Back (trapezius and rhomboids)
◆ Chest (pectoralis major and minor)

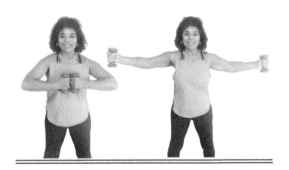

Elbow Side Extensions:

Perform Standing or Seated:

To Begin:

1. Stand with feet shoulder-width apart, feet flat on the floor.

2. Holding small dumbbells in your

hands, your elbows bent, and palms inward on your chest.

3. Straighten your arms to the sides. Return to the starting position and repeat.

4. Complete three sets of 5 to 10 reps. Increase your weight when your strength increases. Wait at least 1-minute in-between sets.

Note: Use light dumbbells of 1 to 2 pounds in the beginning; you can also use any weighted object, such as canned food items or any small, weighted items.

Muscle groups activated by the straight arm pushback:

◆ Shoulders (rear deltoids)
◆ Arms (triceps)
◆ Upper Back (trapezius and rhomboids)

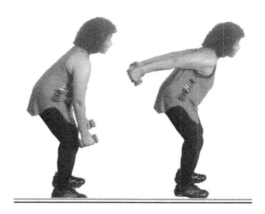

Straight Arm Push Back:

To Begin:

1. Start with your feet, hip distance apart. Engage your abdominals and sit back into a slight squat.

2. Start the dumbbells at the front of the knees. Keeping your core engaged, press the dumbbells past your hips and return with control. Avoid swinging your arms or bending your elbows.

3. Complete three sets of 5 to 10 sets. Increase your weight or sets when your strength increases. Wait at least 1-minute in-between sets.

Note: Use light dumbbells of 1 to 2 pounds in the beginning; you can also use any weighted object, such as canned food items or any small, weighted items.

Lying Down

Muscle groups activated by the lying side lateral raises:

◆   Shoulders (anterior and medial deltoid)

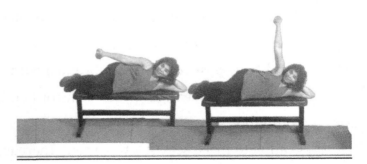

Lying Downside Lateral Raises:

Perform Lying Down, Standing, and Seated

To Begin:

1. Lie on your left side on the floor or on a flat bench with a small dumbbell in your right hand.
2. Start with the dumbbell extended on your thigh.
3. Raise your right arm upwards until it is almost vertical to the floor.
4. Lower your right arm and repeat with the left arm.
5. Keep your spine neutral by supporting your head with your hand.
6. Do not swing your arms up; raise them slowly.
7. Complete three sets of 5 to 10 reps, increase your weight or reps when your strength increases. Wait at least 1-minute in-between sets.

Note: Use light dumbbells of 1 to 2 pounds in the beginning; you can also use any weighted object, such as canned food items or any small, weighted items.

———————————————————

Muscle groups activated by the lying down shoulder press:

- ◆ Shoulders (rear deltoids)
- ◆ Upper Back (trapezius and rhomboids)
- ◆ Lower Back (latissimus dorsi)

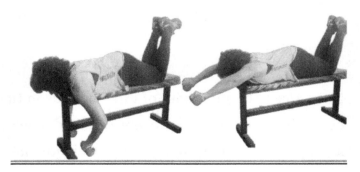

Lying Down Shoulder Press:

Perform Lying Down, Seated or Standing:

To Begin:

1. Lie on your stomach on a flat bench with your chin tucked and arms straight.
2. Reach down, grab the dumbbells, and rotate at the shoulders with the back of the hands facing forward.
3. Take a deep breath and press the dumbbells forward by extending the elbows and contracting the deltoids.
4. Slowly lower the dumbbells back to the starting position (the arms should be roughly 90 degrees or slightly lower depending upon limb lengths).
5. Complete three sets of 5 to 10 reps.
6. Increase your weight or reps when your strength increases. Wait at least 1-minute in-between sets.

Note: Use light dumbbells of 1 to 2 pounds in the beginning; you can also use any weighted object, such as canned food items or any small, weighted items.

_____

Muscle groups activated by the lying down dumbbell pullover:

◆ Shoulders (anterior deltoids)
◆ Chest (pectoralis major and minor)
◆ Abdominal muscles
◆ Upper Back (trapezius and rhomboids)
◆ Lower Back (latissimus dorsi)
◆ Arms (triceps)

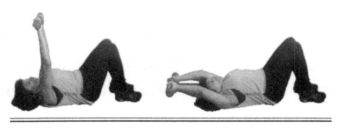

Lying Down Dumbbell Pullover:

Perform Lying Down, Seated or Standing:

To Begin:

1. Lying on your back, grasp a small dumbbell, one in each hand, shoulder-width apart.

2. Lift the dumbbells with arms straight as high as you can.

3. With your arms extended, lower the dumbbells straight back with your elbows locked without

touching the floor.

4. Return to the starting position and repeat.

5. Complete three sets of 5 to 10 reps.

6. Increase your weight or sets when your strength increases. Wait at least 1-minute in-between sets.

Note: Use light dumbbells of 1 to 2 pounds in the beginning; you can also use any weighted object, such as canned food items or any small, weighted items. This exercise can be performed with a weighted barbell for an added challenge.

Muscle groups activated by the lying down rear deltoids fly:

◆   Shoulders (Rear Deltoids)
◆   Upper Back (trapezius and rhomboids)
◆   Lower Back (latissimus dorsi)

105

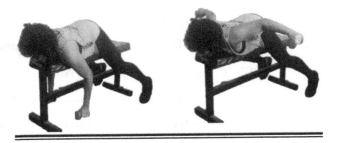

Lying down Rear Deltoids Fly:

To Begin:

1. Lie on a bench, chest facing down, with a small dumbbell in each hand underneath your shoulders.

2. Slightly bend your elbows and raise your arms to the side until they align with your body.

3. Lower the dumbbells to the floor and repeat.

4. Complete three sets of 5 to 10 reps, increase your weight or sets when your strength increases. Wait at least 1-minute in-between sets.

Note: Use light dumbbells of 1 to 2 pounds in the beginning; you can also use any weighted object, such as canned food items or any small, weighted items.

CHEST

The Benefits of Strengthening the Chest

Strengthening the chest is a great way to keep your upper body strong. It will help with everyday tasks and can even help with age-related atrophy. It will also improve your athletic performance and your confidence. Strengthened chest muscles are crucial to a strong upper body. By performing regular chest exercises, you will build up your chest muscles and the rest of your upper body. Deeper breathing exercises are effective in strengthening the chest and diaphragm. They also increase the stability of the core muscles. They also reduce the risk of injuries associated with exercise. Deep breathing exercises help the body breathe more slowly, which can help reduce stress and anxiety.

Strengthening your chest will make it easier to maintain proper posture. Proper posture will improve overall health and reduce pain. Regularly assessing your posture can help you pinpoint any movement problems you may be experiencing.   Proper posture can also prevent injury. Good posture will help you maintain a good range of motion, minimize muscle pain, and make you more flexible and mobile. Muscle atrophy can be caused by a variety of factors, including age. In many cases, muscle atrophy can be reversed through proper nutrition and regular exercise. Increasing strength in the chest of seniors can help them improve their athletic performance. This is because the muscles in the chest are among the largest muscles in the body. They are made up of two types of muscle groups, the pectoralis major and minor.

The pectoralis major helps bend the shoulder joint and pulls the arm toward the chest, while the pectoralis minor pulls the shoulder joint forward and down. Chest muscles also play a role in pushing heavy objects. Moreover, strong chest muscles improve throwing ability. Remember to check with your doctor before beginning any new workout program to ensure any condition you may have is not affected negatively by a particular exercise. Strengthening the chest improves posture and reduces the risk of falling. It also improves balance and stability, making daily life much more enjoyable.

Illustrated Chest Strengthening Exercises

Seated

Muscle groups activated by the seated incline dumbbell press:

◆ Chest (pectoralis major)

◆ Arms (Triceps)
◆ Shoulders (anterior deltoids)

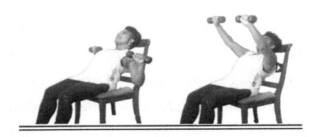

Seated Incline Dumbbell Press:

To Begin:

1. Sit upright comfortably in a good spinal position, shoulders back and Relaxed, looking straight ahead.

2. Grab a small dumbbell in each hand and move towards the front of the chair, leaning back to rest your back, keeping your lower back straight, with your feet flat on the floor.

3. Move both dumbbells up to shoulder level and press the weight towards the ceiling, extend both arms overhead without locking out your elbows, return to the starting position, and

repeat.

4. Complete 5 to 10 reps with three sets, depending on your physical ability. As your strength increases, you can add more weight or extend your reps.

5. Increase your weight when your strength increases. Wait at least 1-minute in-between sets.

Note: Use light dumbbells of 1 to 2 pounds in the beginning; you can also use any weighted object, such as canned food items or any small, weighted items.

Muscle groups activated by the seated incline dumbbell fly:

◆ Chest (pectoralis major)
◆ Shoulders (anterior deltoids)
◆ Arms (Triceps)

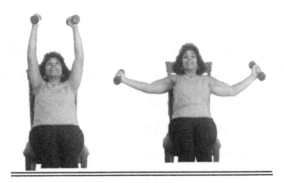

Seated Incline Dumbbell Fly:

To Begin:

1. Sitting on the front of your chair, grab two dumbbells, move towards the front of the chair, keeping your lower back straight, leaning back on the chair.

2. Move both dumbbells up to the top of your chest and stretch both arms towards the ceiling without locking out your elbow.

3. Keep your lower back straight, with your feet flat on the floor.

4. With your arms up towards the ceiling, stretch both arms out until they are parallel with the shoulders.

5. Complete three sets of 5 to 10 reps, increase

your weight or sets when your strength increases. Wait at least 1-minute in-between sets.

Note: Use light dumbbells of 1 to 2 pounds in the beginning; you can also use any weighted object, such as canned food items or any small, weighted items.

Muscle groups activated by the seated chest press with resistance bands:

◆ Arms (biceps and triceps)
◆ Shoulders (anterior deltoids)
◆ Chest (pectoralis major)

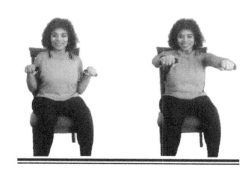

Seated Chest Press with Resistance Bands:

To Begin:

1. Wrap a resistance band around the back of your chair, pulling the band under the armpits and holding the handles in each hand.
2. Sit very tall with your abdominal muscles engaged and begin the movement with the elbows at 90 degrees and at shoulder level with the palms facing down.
3. Squeeze the chest to push the arms straight out in front of you without locking the joints.
4. Bring the arms back to start, keeping the move slow and controlled.
5. You can wrap the band around your hands if you need more tension.
6. Complete three sets of 5 to 10 reps; increase your band tension or reps when your strength increases. Wait at least 1-minute in-between sets.

Standing

Muscle groups activated by the standing chest fly:

- Chest (pectoralis major)
- Shoulders (anterior deltoids)

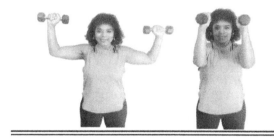

Standing Chest Fly:

Perform Standing or Seated:

To Begin:

1. Stand with your feet shoulder-width apart, your arms out to the sides, holding a small dumbbell in each hand.
2. With your palms facing forward and your

115

elbows directly under your wrists, raise the dumbbells until your upper arms are parallel to the floor.

3 . Bring your elbows and forearms toward the midline of the body and then return to the starting position.

4 . Breathe out as you bring your elbows and forearms toward the body's mid-line and squeeze the chest.

5 . Relax your chest, maintain your upper arms parallel to the floor, and keep your arms at a 90-degree angle.

6 . The movement should only happen at the shoulder joint.

7 . Complete three sets of 5 to 10 reps. Increase your weight or sets when your strength increases. Wait at least 1-minute in-between sets.

Note: Use light dumbbells of 1 to 2 pounds in the beginning; you can also use any weighted object, such as canned food items or any small, weighted items.

Muscle groups activated by the plate press out:

◆ Chest (pectoralis major and minor)
◆ Shoulders (anterior deltoids)
◆ Arms (triceps)
◆ Upper Back (trapezius and rhomboids)

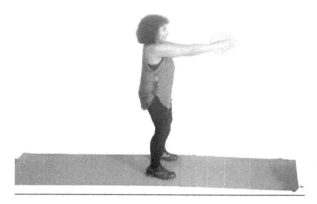

Plate Press Out:

Perform Standing or Seated:

To Begin:

1. Hold a pair of lightweight plates pressing inward between your palms right in front of your chest.

2. Squeeze the plates or dumbbells together, focusing on your chest, and press them out in

front of you until your arms are extended.

3. Flare your lats and pull the weights back to your chest.

4. Complete your reps, and then, on the second set, press the weights downward from your chest at a 45-degree angle.

5. Press them upward at a 45-degree angle on the third set.

6. Increase your weight or sets when your strength increases. Wait at least 1-minute in-between sets.

———————————————

Muscle groups activated by the one-arm hang snatch:

◆ Chest (pectoralis major)
◆ Shoulders (anterior deltoid)
◆ Upper Back (trapezius and rhomboids)
◆ Legs (hamstrings and hips)

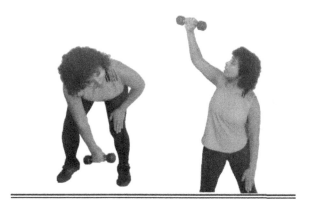

One-Arm Hang Snatch:

To Begin:

1. Stand with feet shoulder-width apart while holding a small dumbbell straight down in front of you. Keeping your back flat and chest up, push your hips back and down to lower the weight between your knees.

2. Explode in one motion, extending the hips quickly and pulling the dumbbell straight up. When the weight reaches maximum height, drop your body underneath, and catch it overhead. Lower back to the starting position, and repeat, switch sides after all reps.

3. Complete three sets of 5 to 10 reps alternating sides.

4 . Increase your weight or sets when your strength increases. Wait at least 1-minute in-between sets.

Note: Use light dumbbells of 1 to 2 pounds in the beginning; you can also use any weighted object, such as canned food items or any small, weighted items.

Muscle groups activated by the standing resistance band press:

◆ Chest (pectoralis major)
◆ Shoulders (anterior deltoid)

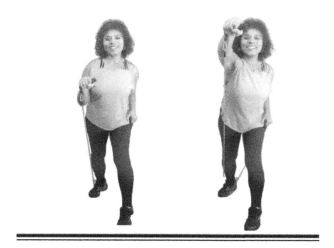

Standing Resistance Band Press:

To Begin:

1. Stand on the band with the heel of your right foot and step forward with your left foot.
2. Take the band and press out and up to work the upper chest. Be careful not to push straight up. It should be at an angle.
3. Complete three sets of 5 to 10 reps. Increase your ban tension when your strength increases. Wait at least 1-minute in-between sets.

Lying Down

Muscle groups activated by the dumbbell chest fly:

- ◆ Chest (pectoralis major)
- ◆ Shoulders (anterior deltoids)
- ◆ Arms (biceps)

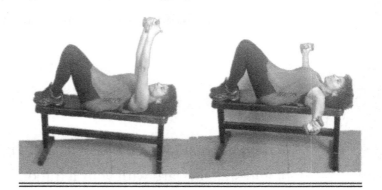

Dumbbell Chest Fly:

To Begin:

1. Lie flat on your back on a flat bench holding two small dumbbells with your arms extended, palms facing inward, without locking out the elbows.

122

Place your feet firmly on top of the bench as illustrated or on the floor on either side of the bench.

2 . Inhale and slowly lower the dumbbells in an arc motion until they align with the chest. Your arms will be extended to the sides with the elbow not locked. Do not drop your arms lower than your shoulders.

3 . Exhale and slowly press the dumbbells up in the same arc motion.

4 . Complete at least three sets of 5 to 10 reps. Increase your weight or sets when your strength increases. Wait at least 1-minute in-between sets.

Note: Use light dumbbells of 1 to 2 pounds in the beginning; you can also use any weighted object, such as canned food items or any small, weighted items.

Muscle groups activated by the floor dumbbell chest press:

◆   Chest (pectoralis major and minor)

◆　Shoulders (anterior, medial, posterior deltoids)

◆　Arms (triceps)

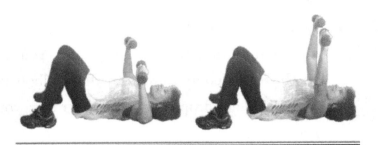

Floor Dumbbell Chest Press:

To Begin:

1. Lie flat on your back with your knees up and your feet flat on the floor.

2. Hold a small dumbbell in each hand above your chest.

3. Extend your arms toward the ceiling without locking out your elbows and return to the starting position and repeat.

4. Your goal is three sets of 5 to 10 reps depending on your physical ability.

5. As you get stronger, increase your weight, reps, sets, or both.

6. Wait at least 1-minute in-between sets.

Note: Use light dumbbells of 1 to 2 pounds in the beginning; you can also use any weighted object, such as canned food items or any small, weighted items.

Muscle groups activated by the lying down dumbbell pullover:

- Chest (Pectoralis Major and Minor)
- Shoulders (anterior deltoid)
- Abdominal muscles
- Upper Back (trapezius and rhomboids)
- Lower Back (latissimus dorsi)
- Arms (Triceps)

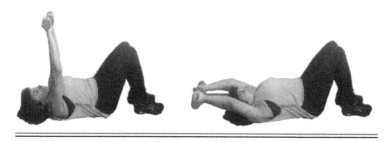

Lying Down Dumbbell Pullover:

Perform Lying Down, Seated or Standing:

To Begin:

1. Lie on your back on the floor and hold two small dumbbells overhead, one in each hand.
2. Press the weight over your chest, then reach back over your head, bending your elbows slightly.
3. Continue until you feel a stretch in your lats, then pull the dumbbell back over your chest.
4. Take a deep breath when you lower the dumbbell behind you.
5. Complete three sets of 5 to 10 reps. Increase your weight or your sets when your strength increases. Wait at least 1-minute in-between sets.

Note: Use light dumbbells of 1 to 2 pounds in the beginning; you can also use any weighted object, such as canned food items or any small, weighted items.

Muscle groups activated by the half-body push-ups:

◆ Chest (pectoralis major)

◆ Arms (biceps and triceps)
◆ Shoulders (anterior deltoids)

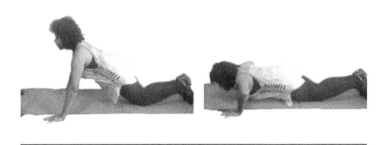

Half Body Push-Ups:

To Begin:

Get into a half-body push-up position: knees on the floor with hands under your shoulders.

1. Your entire body should be straight and your core braced.
2. Lower your body, keeping your head neutral until your chest almost touches the floor.
3. Fire your chest and triceps and raise your body back to the push-up position.
4. Complete three sets of 5 to 10 push-ups. Increase your reps, sets or both when your strength increases. Wait at least 1-minute between sets.

BICEPS

The Benefits of Strengthening the Biceps

As we age, our bodies begin to lose muscle mass. Even seniors who stay in shape may notice increased muscle weakness as they age. Muscle mass decreases by roughly 3-8% per decade after age 30 and even higher after age 60. By age 80, the percentage is more than two-thirds. Regular exercise is a great way to maintain muscle tone. Exercise can help seniors with arm weakness by allowing them to keep the strength of their arms. For older adults, weightlifting exercises can improve arm strength.

These exercises can be performed seated or standing, with some exercises lying down. Exercises for the arm are essential for aging adults with limited mobility. They can improve arm strength and flexibility while reducing the pain caused by arthritis. Exercise can also improve joint flexibility and help relieve joint pain and mobility. Proper form is essential when exercising the biceps. The illustrations shown in this book will guide you through the proper technique to use. Before starting an exercise program, it is essential to get medical clearance. Ask about activities that could worsen preexisting conditions and ask about safe and inadvisable exercises because everyone's situation and fitness level are different. It is also essential to consider whether you have any ongoing health issues. For example, if you have diabetes, you may need to adjust your meal plans or timing of medications.

Physical activity is beneficial for your health, both physically and mentally. If you are not used to exercising, starting slowly and building up from there is essential. It is possible to get injured and stop exercising altogether if you start too quickly. To avoid injuries, a slow and steady approach is best. Begin with low-intensity exercises and gradually increase your intensity as you feel more comfortable. Always warm up before exercising and pay attention to your surroundings, especially outdoors. Drinking water before, during, and after a workout is also recommended. Even if you are not thirsty, drink water to stay hydrated.

Illustrated Biceps Strengthening Exercises

Seated

Muscle groups activated by the seated barbell bicep curl:

◆ Arms (biceps, triceps and forearms, and wrist)

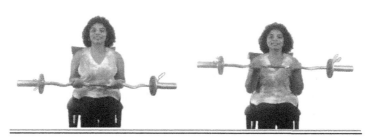

Seated Barbell Biceps Curl:

Perform Seated or Standing:

To Begin:

1. Place weights on your barbell that is comfortable for your physical ability.
2. Sit upright comfortably in a good spinal position, shoulders back and Relaxed, looking straight ahead.
3. Hold the barbell waist high while sitting and slowly lift the barbell towards the top of your

chest without resting at the top; only hinge from the elbows and not the shoulders.

4. Slowly return to the starting position and repeat

5. Complete three sets of 5 to 10 reps; increase your weight or reps as your body strengthens.

6. Wait at least 1-minute in-between sets.

Muscle groups activated by the seated alternating dumbbell bicep curl:

◆   Arms (biceps, triceps, forearms, and wrist)

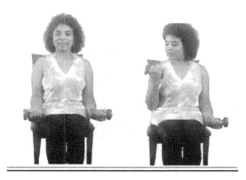

Seated Alternating Dumbbell Biceps Curl:

Perform Seated or Standing:

To Begin:

1. Sit upright comfortably in a good spinal position, shoulders back and Relaxed, with a small dumbbell in each hand.
2. Slowly lift the dumbbell in your right hand up past your chest and toward your shoulders, hinging only at the elbow. Your upper arm should not move. At the top of the movement, pause to squeeze your biceps muscles.
3. Repeat the movement alternating with your left hand.
4. Complete three sets of 5 to 10 reps, bending only at the elbows. Increase your weight or reps as your strength level increases. Wait at least 1-minute in-between sets.

Note: Use light dumbbells of 1 to 2 pounds in the beginning; you can also use any weighted object, such as canned food items or any small, weighted items.

Muscle groups activated by the seated one-arm biceps curl:

◆   Arms (biceps, triceps, forearms, and wrist)

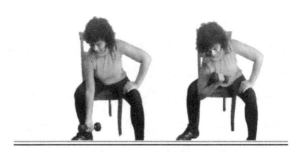

Seated One-Arm Biceps Curl:

Perform Seated or Standing:

To Begin:

1. Grab a small dumbbell with your right hand. Rest your right upper arm against the upper part of the thigh. Rotate the wrist so your palm faces forward, away from your thigh. Your arm should be extended, and the dumbbell should be above the floor. This will be your starting position.
2. Curl the dumbbell upward while contracting the biceps as you breathe out. Only the forearms

should move. Continue the movement until your biceps are fully contracted, and the dumbbell is at shoulder level.

3. Hold the position while contracting the biceps muscle.

4. Slowly bring the dumbbells back to starting position as you breathe in.

5. Complete three sets of 5 to 10 reps alternating to your left arm.

6. Increase your weight or reps when your strength increases. Wait at least 1-minute in-between sets.

Note: Use light dumbbells of 1 to 2 pounds in the beginning; you can also use any weighted object, such as canned food items or any small, weighted items.

_____

Standing

Muscle groups activated by the standing barbell bicep curl:

◆ Arms (biceps, triceps, forearms, and wrist)

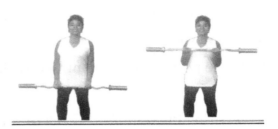

Standing Barbell Biceps Curl:

Perform Standing or Seated:

To Begin:

1. Load an appropriate amount of weight onto a barbell that you can lift for 5-10 reps.
2. Grab the barbell tightly with a shoulder-width underhand grip.
3. Stand up straight with the bar resting on your thighs. Your chest should be up, and your shoulders pinned back slightly.
4. Curl the bar toward your shoulders by flexing your biceps, bending only at the elbow joint.
5. Keep lifting before the undersides of your forearms reach the biceps. In other words, do

not bring the bar all the way up; leave just a slight tension before the very top.

6. Hold the contraction for a second and lower the weight under control back down without locking out the elbows.

7. Perform three sets of 5 to 10 reps. Increase your weight or sets when your strength increases. Wait at least 1-minute in-between sets.

Muscle groups activated by the side biceps curl with resistance bands:

◆ Arms (biceps, triceps, forearms, and wrist)
◆ Shoulders (anterior deltoids)

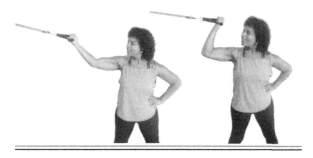

Side Biceps Curl with Resistance Bands:

137

To Begin:

1. Secure the band(s) to the door with the door anchor firmly in place.
2. Attach both ends of the band(s) to one handle and grip the handle with one hand.
3. Stand with your side to the door (the side with the active arm) far enough away from the door so that the band starts to stretch when your arm is up.
4. Your active arm should be straight, parallel to the floor, and palm up, with a slight bend at the elbow with your inactive hand on your hip.
5. Pull the handle and bend your arm until your hand is above your upper arm.
6. Complete three sets of 5 to 10 reps. Increase your band tension when your strength increases. Wait at least 1-minute in-between sets.

Muscle groups activated by the standing dumbbell biceps curl:

◆   Arms (biceps, triceps, forearms, and wrist)

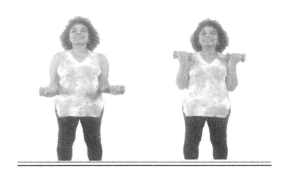

Standing Dumbbell Biceps Curl:

Perform Standing or Seated:

To Begin:

After picking up a small dumbbell in each hand, stand with your feet shoulder-width apart, with your arms at your sides and palms facing away from your body.

1. Lift the dumbbells waist high, keeping your elbows close to your body, and curl the dumbbells bending at the elbow, curling up

towards the shoulder, hinging only at the elbow.

2. Hold for one second and slowly lower your arms to return to the starting position.

3. Repeat this movement 5 to 10 times for three sets. Increase your weight or sets when your strength increases. Wait at least 1-minute in-between sets.

Note: Use light dumbbells of 1 to 2 pounds in the beginning; you can also use any weighted object, such as canned food items or any small, weighted items.

Muscle groups activated by the one-arm preacher curl with resistance bands:

◆ Arms (biceps, triceps, forearms, and wrist)

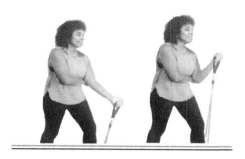

One Arm Preacher Curls with Resistance Band:

Perform Standing or Seated:

To Begin:

1. Keep your back flat, your head straight, and your chest up.
2. Position your non-active arm across your body, with the back of your non-active hand stabilizing your active elbow.
3. Your active arm should be almost straight (there should still be a slight bend at the elbow) with your palms facing forward.
4. Pull the handle(s) and bend your arm at the elbow until your hand is at chest height.
5. Complete three sets of 5 to 10 reps. Increase your band tension when your strength

increases. Wait at least 1-minute in-between sets.

Lying Down

Muscle groups activated by the lying down biceps curl:

◆   Arms (biceps, triceps, forearms, and wrist)

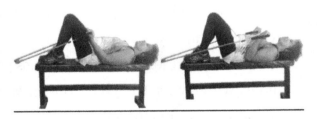

Lying Down Biceps Curl:

Perform Lying Down, Standing, or Seated:

To Begin:

1.   Secure the band(s) to the door with the door anchor at the bottom of the door.

2.   Attach each end of the band(s) to a handle.

3. Grip a handle in each hand and lay on your back with your feet 1 to 2 feet away from the door. Your knees should be up and your feet flat on the flat bench or floor.

4. Start with your arms straight and tight to your body with palms facing up.

5. Pull the handles and bend your arms until your hands are directly over your chest, be careful not to rest your elbows on the bench or the floor.

6. Complete three sets of 5 to 10 reps. Wait at least 1-minute in-between sets.

7. Increase your band tension when your strength increases. Wait at least 1-minute in-between sets.

Muscle groups activated by the lying down biceps curl with bands with arms up:

◆ Arms (biceps, triceps, forearms, and wrist)
◆ Upper Back (trapezius and rhomboids)

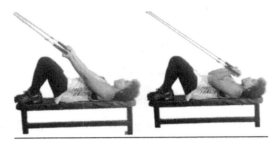

Lying Down Biceps Curl with Resistance Bands with Arms Up:

To Begin:

1. Secure the band(s) to the door with the door anchor at the top of the door.
2. Attach each end of the band(s) to a handle.
3. Grab a handle with each hand and lay on the floor or a bench with your knees bent, your feet flat on the floor or bench, and your toes touching the door.
4. Your arms should be straight, pointed towards the door anchor, with your palms facing up.
5. Pull the handles down and bend your arms until your hands are right in front of your face.
6. Complete three sets of 5 to 10 reps and wait at least 1-minute in-between sets.
7. Increase your band tension when your strength

increases. Wait at least 1-minute in-between sets.

———————————

Muscle groups activated by the lying down dumbbell biceps curl:

◆　Arms (biceps, triceps, forearms, and wrist)

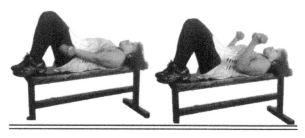

Lying Down Dumbbell Bicep Curl:

Perform Lying Down, Seated or Standing:

To Begin:

1. Grab a pair of light dumbbells with an underhand grip.
2. Lie back on a weight bench.
3. Keep your elbows parallel to the bench without resting the elbows on the bench.

4. Curl the weights with control toward your front delts.

5. Keep lifting until your forearms and biceps almost touch.

6. Slowly lower the dumbbells until your elbows are completely extended.

7. Repeat for three sets of 5-10 reps; wait for at least 1-minute in-between sets.

8. Increase your weight or reps when your strength increases. Wait at least 1-minute in-between sets.

Note: Use light dumbbells of 1 to 2 pounds in the beginning; you can also use any weighted object, such as canned food items or any small, weighted items.

TRICEPS

The Benefits of Strengthening the Triceps

The benefits of strengthening the triceps are numerous. In addition to being necessary for daily tasks such as lifting groceries and pulling laundry, they also help maintain your body's joint stability. They improve your range of motion and boost your metabolism, so you burn more calories.

The triceps are a muscle located in the back of the upper arm. They are essential for everyday activities, such as extending the elbow, lifting heavy objects, and throwing. They have more fast-twitch muscle fibers than slow-twitch fibers. These fibers are better for endurance activities, but they fatigue more quickly. Strengthening the triceps is essential for seniors. It can prevent injuries, such as broken bones, and it can increase the time seniors can enjoy activities they enjoy. They also increase bone density, which can decrease the risk of osteoporosis.

Illustrated Triceps Strengthening Exercises

Seated

Muscle groups activated by the seated triceps kick-back:

◆   Arms (triceps)

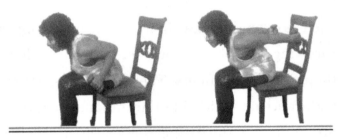

Seated Triceps Kick-back:
Perform Seated or Standing:

To Begin:

1. Sit on the end of a bench or chair while holding a small dumbbell in each hand.
2. Bend your torso over with your back straight.

3. Then lift your elbows up so they are tucked into your sides with your upper arms parallel to the floor.

4. Slowly extend your forearms behind you so your arms are parallel to the floor.

5. Contract your triceps and hold for a couple of seconds.

6. Bring your forearms back down so they are at a 90-degree angle to your upper arms.

7. Complete three sets of 5 to 10 reps; increase your weight or reps when your strength increases. Wait at least 1-minute in-between sets.

Note: Use light dumbbells of 1 to 2 pounds in the beginning; you can also use any weighted object, such as canned food items or any small, weighted items.

-

Muscle groups activated by the seated overhead triceps extension:

- Arms (triceps)
- Shoulders (anterior deltoids, posterior deltoids)
- Abdominal muscles

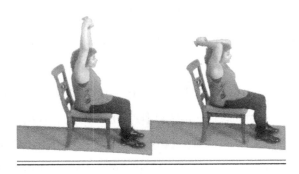

Seated Overhead Triceps Extension:

Perform Seated or Standing:

To Begin:

1. Sit with your feet shoulder-width apart, with your arms extended, holding a small dumbbell with both hands over your head.

2. With your upper arm stationary and bending only at the elbow, lower the dumbbell until your forearm is parallel to the floor, squeeze your triceps, and raise the dumbbell back to the starting position without locking out the elbow.

3 .   Repeat this movement for three sets of 5 to 10 reps; increase your weight or sets when your strength increases. Wait at least 1-minute in-between sets.

Note: Use light dumbbells of 1 to 2 pounds in the beginning; you can also use any weighted object, such as canned food items or any small, weighted items.

Muscle groups activated by the seated alternating overhead triceps extension:

◆   Arms (triceps)
◆   Shoulders (anterior deltoids, posterior deltoids)
◆   Abdominal muscles

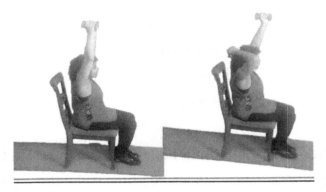

Seated Alternating Overhead Triceps Extension:

Perform Seated or Standing:

To Begin:

1. Sit with your feet shoulder-width apart, holding a small dumbbell in each hand.
2. With your upper arm stationary and bending only at the elbow, lower your right arm until your forearm is parallel to the floor, squeeze your triceps, and raise the dumbbell back to the starting position without locking out the elbow. Repeat with the left arm.
3. Repeat this movement for 5 to 10 reps for three sets.
4. Increase your weight or sets when your

strength increases. Wait at least 1-minute in-between sets.

Note: Use light dumbbells of 1 to 2 pounds in the beginning; you can also use any weighted object, such as canned food items or any small, weighted items.

Muscle groups activated by the seated resistance band overhead triceps extension:

- Arms (triceps)
- Shoulders (anterior deltoids, posterior deltoids)
- Abdominal muscles

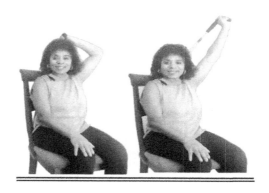

Seated Resistance Band Overhead Triceps Extension:

To Begin:
1. Sit with your right foot on one end of the exercise band and loop it around the back of the chair and over your left shoulder.
2. Hold the other end in the left hand, behind your head.
3. Keep the shoulders relaxed, then extend the left arm towards the ceiling without locking out the elbows.
4. Lower your arm behind your head, ensuring your forearm goes no further than parallel to the floor.
5. Repeat for the left arm.
6. Complete three sets of 5 to 10 reps alternating arms. Increase your band tension when your strength increases. Wait at least 1-minute in-between sets.

_____

Standing

Muscle groups activated by the triceps dips:

- Arms (triceps and biceps)
- Chest (pectoralis major)
- Shoulders (anterior deltoids, posterior deltoids)

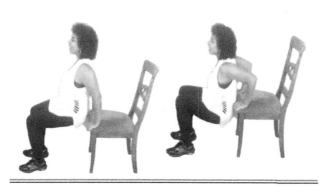

Triceps Dips:

To Begin:

1. Sit on a chair or bench with your hands just outside the hips, with your knees bent.
2. Lift onto the hands and, keeping the glutes and

lower back very close to the chair or bench, bend your elbows, lowering down until they're at about 90 degrees.

3. Keep your elbows pointing behind you, the shoulders down, and the abdominal muscles engaged.

4. Push back to start and repeat for three sets of 5 to 10 reps. Increase your reps, sets or both when your strength increases. Wait at least 1-minute in-between sets.

Muscle groups activated by the resistance band triceps extension:

◆ Arms (triceps)
◆ Shoulders (anterior deltoids, medial deltoids)
◆ Abdominal muscles

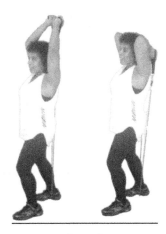

Resistance Band Triceps Extension:

To Begin:

1. Stand with one foot slightly in front of the other and place the center of the band under the back foot.
2. Bring handles together above your head without locking out the elbows.
3. Slowly lower handles behind the back of your head until elbows are bent 90 degrees.
4. Keep your elbows close to the side of your head.
5. Press hands back up overhead slowly.
6. Complete three sets of 5 to 10 reps, increase

your reps, sets or both when your strength increases. Wait at least 1-minute in-between sets.

Muscle groups activated by the triceps kick-back:

◆   Arms (triceps)

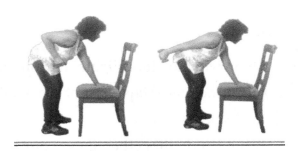

Triceps Kick-Back:

Perform Standing or Seated:

To Begin:

1.   With a small dumbbell in hand, place your other hand on the chair seat for support. This could be any stable item to enable you to bend

at the waist and offer support.

2 . Bring your upper arm close to your body and firmly hold it against your body.

3 . Bending only at the elbow joint, push the dumbbell back, and return to the start.

4 . Complete three sets of 5 to 10 reps alternating arms. Increase your weight or sets when your strength increases. Wait at least 1-minute in-between sets.

Note: Use light dumbbells of 1 to 2 pounds in the beginning; you can also use any weighted object, such as canned food items or any small, weighted items.

Muscle groups activated by the triceps extension:

◆ Arms (triceps)
◆ Shoulders (anterior deltoids, medial deltoid)
◆ Abdominal muscles

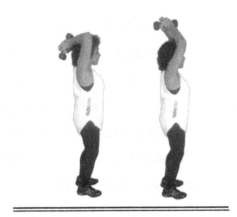

Standing Dumbbell Triceps Extension:

Perform Standing or Seated:

To Begin:

1. Stand tall and hold a small dumbbell with both hands directly above your head.
2. Slowly raise your arms, bending only at the elbows above your head as you keep your upper arms fixed alongside your head, keeping your elbows slightly bent.
3. Extend your arms and repeat.
4. Complete three sets of 5 to 10 reps; increase your weight or reps when your strength increases. Wait at least 1-minute in-between

sets.

Note: Use light dumbbells of 1 to 2 pounds in the beginning; you can also use any weighted object, such as canned food items or any small, weighted items.

Lying Down

Muscle groups activated by the alternating dumbbell triceps extension:

♦ Arms (triceps)
♦ Shoulder Joint stabilization

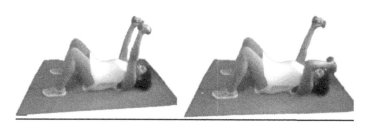

Alternating Dumbbell Triceps Extension:

Perform Lying Down, Seated or Standing:

To Begin:

1. Lying back on a bench or the floor, with a small dumbbell in each hand, your arms fully extended overhead.

2. Keeping one dumbbell stationary, lower the other by bending at the elbow until it is just above your shoulder.

3. Pause, then extend the arm back to the start position by contracting the triceps.

4. Complete three sets of 5 to 10 reps. Increase your weight or sets when your strength increases. Wait at least 1-minute in-between sets.

Note: Use light dumbbells of 1 to 2 pounds in the beginning; you can also use any weighted object, such as canned food items or any small, weighted items.

_____

Muscle groups activated by the dumbbell triceps extension:

◆ Arms (triceps)

◆ Shoulder Joint stabilization

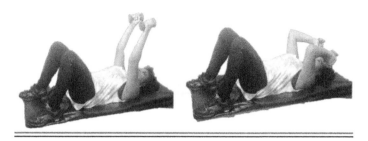

Dumbbell Triceps Extension:

Perform Lying Down, Seated or Standing:

To Begin:

1. Lie on a bench on the floor, and hold a small dumbbell in each hand, extended overhead without locking out the elbows.
2. Move both dumbbells down, only flexing at the elbows until your forearms are parallel to the floor.
3. Extend the arm upward to the starting position without locking out the elbows.
4. Complete 5 to 10 reps; increase your weight or sets when your strength increases. Wait at least 1-minute in-between sets.

Note: Use light dumbbells of 1 to 2 pounds in the beginning; you can also use any weighted object, such as canned food items or any small, weighted items.

_____

Muscle groups activated by the knee push-up:

◆   Chest (pectoralis major and minor)
◆   Arms (biceps and triceps)
◆   Shoulders (anterior deltoids)

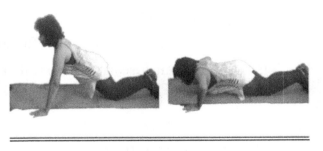

Knee Push-Ups:

To Begin:

1. Get into a half-body push-up position which is knees on the floor with hands under your shoulders.
2. Your entire body should be straight, and your Abdominal muscles braced.
3. Lower your body, keeping your head neutral until your chest almost touches the floor.
4. Fire your chest and triceps and raise your body back to the push-up position.
5. Complete 5 to 10 push-ups three times. Increase your reps, sets or both when your strength increases. Wait at least 1-minute in-between sets.

Muscle groups activated by the lying down band triceps extension:

- Arms (triceps)
- Shoulders (anterior deltoids)
- Abdominal muscles

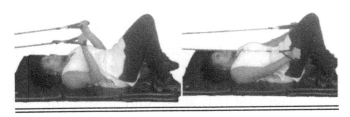

Lying Down Band Triceps Extension:

To Begin:

1. Secure the band to the door with the door anchor at the bottom of the door.

2. Attach a handle to each end of the band and grip them with each hand.

3. Your fingers should be inside the handle, and your thumb on the outside.

4. Lay on the floor with your body facing away from the door and your head about 2 to 3 feet away from the door.

5. Keep your knees bent and together, feet flat on the floor, and elbows tight to your side.

6. Start with your arms bent, hands directly over your chest, and palms facing forward.

7. Push the handles out towards your feet, straightening your arms.

8 . Complete three sets of 5 to 10 reps. Increase your band tension when your strength increases. Wait at least 1-minute in-between sets.

FOREARMS and WRISTS

The Benefits of Strengthening the Forearms and Wrists

A strong forearm and wrist will help you strengthen your grip and reduce inflammation in your joints. These illustrated exercises can also improve overall strength and flexibility. They are recommended as part of a daily routine. They are also recommended for people who engage in strenuous activity.

These exercises are designed to target specific muscles in the forearm. They can be performed alone or in conjunction with a more strenuous exercise routine.

Performing these exercises in a controlled manner will help you benefit most from them. Increasing grip strength should be an essential element of achieving your goals. You will find it easier to lift objects, open bottles, and open doors with it. The illustrations in this chapter will help improve your grip strength, although you should be careful not to overdo them. The best exercise to increase grip strength is strengthening your forearms and wrists.

The forearms and wrists are the most underrated muscles in the body. These muscles do much more than make you look stronger. They are responsible for lifting real-world objects, bending things, opening containers, and unlocking doors. The forearm is one of the main parts of your body that you use in most activities. This is the part of your arm between your wrist and the elbow. Wrist and forearm exercises are a way to combat arthritis and osteoporosis.

Illustrated Forearms and Wrists Strengthening Exercises

Seated

Muscle groups activated by the seated dumbbell wrist curl:

◆ Arms (forearms and wrist)
◆ Brachioradialis muscle (located: on the side of the forearm)

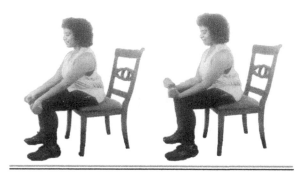

Seated Dumbbell Wrist Curl:
Perform Seated or Standing:

To Begin:

1. Grab two small dumbbells with an underhand grip (palms up) and sit on the end of a bench or chair,

2. Rest your forearms on your thighs, with your wrists hanging off the front of your knees, about 6 to 8 inches apart.

3. Slowly lower the weight by bending your wrists toward the floor. Feel the muscles stretch. Hold for one count.

4. Curl the weight up as high as you can, moving the palms of your hands toward you. Hold this position for a second while contracting the forearm muscle.

5. Then slowly return the dumbbells to the starting position and repeat.

6. Complete three sets of 5 to 10 reps; increase your weight or sets when your strength increases. Wait at least 1-minute in-between sets.

Note: Use light dumbbells of 1 to 2 pounds in the beginning; you can also use any weighted object, such as canned food items or any small, weighted items.

Muscle groups activated by the seated reverse dumbbell wrist curl:

◆ Arms (forearms and wrist)

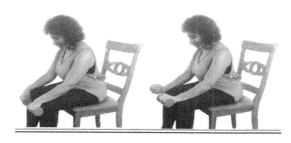

Seated Reverse Dumbbell Wrist Curl:

Perform Seated or Standing:

To Begin:

1. Grab two small dumbbells with an overhand grip (palms down) and sit on the end of a bench or chair,

2. Rest your forearms on your thighs, with your wrists hanging off the front of your knees, about 6 to 8 inches apart.

3. Slowly lower the weight by bending your wrists toward the floor. Feel the muscles stretch. Hold

for one count.

4 . Curl the weight up as high as you can, moving the back of your hands toward you. Hold this position for a second while contracting the forearm muscle.

5 . Then slowly return to the starting position and repeat.

6 . Complete three sets of 5 to 10 reps; increase your weight or sets when your strength increases. Wait at least 1-minute in-between sets.

Note: Use light dumbbells of 1 to 2 pounds initially; you can also use any weighted object, such as canned food items or any small, weighted items.

Muscle groups activated by the dumbbell radial and ulnar deviation:

◆   Arms (forearms and wrist)

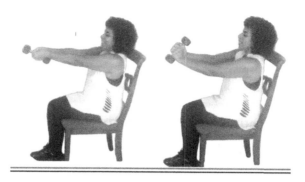

Dumbbell Radial and Ulnar Deviation:

Perform Seated, Standing or Lying Down:

To Begin:

1. Sit and hold one small dumbbell in both hands. Keep your arms extended in front of you.

2. Without bending your elbow, flex your wrist up toward your body. Hold this pose for a second.

3. Slowly lower the wrist so your knuckles point away from your body.

4. Complete three sets of 5 to 10 reps, increase your weight or sets when your strength increases. Wait at least 1-minute in-between sets.

Note: Use light dumbbells of 1 to 2 pounds initially; you can also use any weighted object, such as canned food items or any small, weighted items.

Muscle groups activated by the seated reverse barbell wrist curl:

◆   Arms (forearms and wrist)

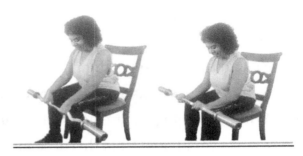

Seated Reverse Barbell Wrist Curl:

Perform Seated or Standing:

To Begin:

1. Grasp a barbell using an overhand grip (palms facing down) and sit down on the end of a flat bench or off the knees while sitting, as shown.

2. Rest the front of your forearms on the top of your thighs or the end of the bench so that your

wrists are off the end of your knees or the bench.

3 . Without moving the forearms, slowly raise your hands as far as possible (bending at the wrist), squeezing the forearm muscles at the top of the movement.

4 . Pause and slowly lower the barbell back to the starting position.

5 . Complete three sets of 5 to 10 reps, increase your weight, and sets when your strength increases. Wait at least 1-minute in-between sets.

Standing

Muscle groups activated by the resistance band wrist curls:

◆   Arms (forearms and wrist)

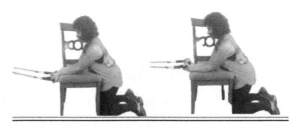

Resistance Band Wrist Curls:

Perform Standing or Seated:

To Begin:

1. Kneel in front of a bench or chair and grab your resistance band handles with your palms facing up.
2. Place your wrist just off the edge of the chair or bench, making sure your bands have good tension,
3. Press the back of your hand toward the floor, bending at the wrist only.
4. Move your hand upward, bending only at the wrist.
5. Complete three sets of 5 to 10 reps; increase your reps, sets or band tension when your strength increases. Wait at least 1-minute in-between sets.

Muscle groups activated by the front wrist rotation:

◆ Arms (forearms and wrist)

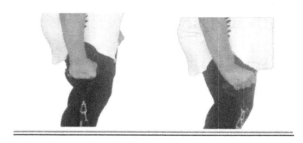

Front wrist Rotation:

Perform Standing, Seated or Lying Down:

To Begin:

1. Place your hands by your sides in a neutral wrist position, elbows fully locked out.
2. Curl the thumb side of your hands up towards your body while keeping the rest of your arms completely still.

3 . Squeeze your forearms for a split second, then lower the bands to the starting point.

4 . Repeat for 2-3 sets of 5-10 reps, increasing band tension when you feel stronger. Wait at least 1-minute in-between sets.

Muscle groups activated by the wrist strengthening stretches:

◆ Arms (wrist)

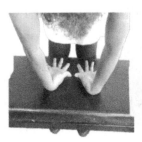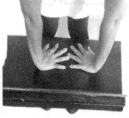

Wrist Strengthening Stretches:

To Begin:

1. Kneel and extend both your hands in front of you and ensure they are shoulder-width apart. Flex your palms so that your fingertips point back toward you.

2. Keeping your wrists flexed, place the back of your palms on the floor or table, apply gentle pressure, and hold this pose for 30 seconds. You can fist your palms and release them while holding this pose.

3. Release the hold after 30 seconds. Extend your wrists and turn your palms down.

4. Place your palms on the floor or table and hold this pose for 30 seconds.

5. Release and shake your hands.

6. Complete this sequence three times. Wait at least 1-minute in-between sets.

———————————————————

Lying Down

Muscle groups activated by the tennis ball squeeze:

- ◆ Arms (forearms and wrist)
- ◆ Hand

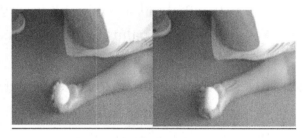

Tennis Ball Squeeze:

Perform Lying Down, Standing, or Seated:

To Begin:

1. Hold a tennis ball with your left hand and place your left forearm on a table.
2. Squeeze the tennis ball and count to five.
3. Release.
4. Complete three sets of 5 to 10 times. Increase your reps, sets or both or sets when your grip

strength gets stronger. Wait at least 1-minute in-between sets.

Muscle groups activated by the lying down wrist circles:

◆ Arms (forearm and wrist)

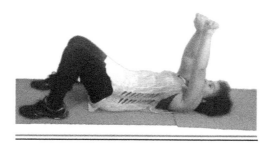

Lying Wrist Circles:

Perform Lying Down, Seated or Standing:

To Begin:

1. Lye with your spine erect, shoulders rolled back, and looking at the ceiling.
2. Extend your hands upward at the shoulder level and fold each palm into a fist.

3. Keeping your elbows stationary, turn your wrists to the left, flex them up, turn to the right, and then flex down. Repeat ten times.

4. Reverse the direction and repeat it ten times.

5. Complete three sets of flexing ten times. Wait at least 1-minute in-between sets.

Time to Rest

"Rest is a productive activity." – Sophia Joan.

We have talked about the importance of knowing when to take a break, and it is with that in mind I'm going to interrupt our flow here for a moment.

Regular strength training is essential for all of us as we age, but it is important to remember that more is not always better – rest is just as crucial in strength-building as the training itself is. During rest periods, your muscles can repair and grow, allowing you to reap the benefits of all the work you are putting in and minimize the risk of injury.

Of course, suppose you are only working on one area of the body per session. In that case, there's no reason you shouldn't strength train on consecutive days – you might, for example, work on your arms on Monday and give them a rest on Tuesday while you work on your legs... or you might do balance exercises one day to give your muscles a chance to recuperate. There is nothing wrong with a complete day of rest, though; you will find it easier to work through the exercises if you take one.

And during *this* moment of rest, before we jump back into the next exercises, I would like to take the opportunity to ask you a favor. Strength training is a vital part of staying fit and healthy as we age, and I want to get this guidance out to as many older adults as I can… and the easiest way to do that is through reviews.

By leaving a review of this book on Amazon, you will show other readers where they can find all the guidance, they need to build their strength safely and embrace their golden years with energy and good health.

Simply by telling new readers how this book has helped you and what they can expect to find within its pages, you'll show other seniors where they can find everything they need to restore their energy, build their strength, and improve their balance and flexibility.

Thank you for your support. Now, let us get back to those exercises!

HANDS

The Benefits of Strengthening the Hands

Hand strengthening exercises can help improve your range of motion in the fingers and thumbs. By strengthening these muscles, you can lift heavier objects. A rubber band exercise is a great way to reinforce the thumbs, illustrated below. Hand strength training is also essential for seniors with problems using their hands. Age-related declines in hand function may affect the muscles that control the thumb. In this case, increasing hand strength could improve their function and assist in independent living.

Dumbbell wrist curls, as illustrated in the forearms and wrist section, can be used to develop strong grips by developing wrist and forearm strength. If you suffer from arthritis, hand stiffness, pain, and weakness, it can limit your ability to do everyday tasks. Hand exercises can improve arthritis symptoms and give you the flexibility to do those daily activities.

Illustrated Hands Strengthening Exercises

Benefits of the thumb extension:

- Strengthens your thumb.
- Increases your range of motion.
- Relieves pain.

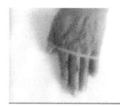 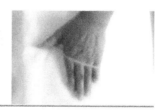

Thumb Extension:

To Begin:

1. Put your hand flat on a table. Wrap a rubber band around your hand at the base of your finger joints.
2. Gently move your thumb away from your fingers as far as possible.

3. Hold for 30 to 60 seconds and release.

4. Repeat 10 to 15 times with both hands. You can do this exercise two to three times a week but rest your hands for 48 hours in between sessions.

Muscle groups activated by the claw stretch:

◆ Greatly improves the range of motion in your fingers.

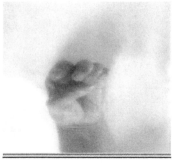

Claw stretch:

To Begin:

1. Hold your hand out in front of you.

2. Bend your fingertips until they touch the base of the finger joints.

3. Hold for 30-60 seconds, then release.

4. Complete three sets, ten reps, with each hand.

Benefits of the thumb flex:

◆ Strengthens your thumb.
◆ Increases your range of motion.
◆ Relieves pain.

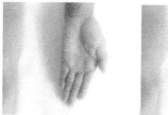 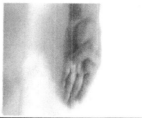

Thumb Flex:

To Begin:

1. Hold your hand out in front of you, palm up.

2. Extend your thumb away from your other fingers as far as possible.

3. Then bend your thumb across your palm to

touch the base of your small finger.

4. Hold for 30 to 60 seconds.

5. Repeat at least four times with both thumbs.

Benefits of the pinch strengthener:

◆ As a physical therapy tool, it will help strengthen the muscles of the hand and wrist.

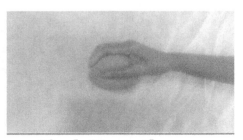

Pinch Strengthener:

To Begin:

1. Pinch a soft foam ball or putty between your fingertips and thumb.

2. Hold for 30 to 60 seconds.

3. Repeat 10 to 15 times on both hands. Do this

/ SENIOR STRENGTH EXERCISES 60+

exercise two to three times a week but rest your hands for 48 hours in between sessions.

THE CORE and ITS FUNCTION

Working out the core for seniors has many benefits, including improved posture, better movement control, and lessening the risk of injuries. Core muscles include the transverse abdominis, multifidus, internal and external obliques, erector spinae, diaphragm, pelvic floor muscles, and the rectus abdominis (Abdominal muscles). The minor core consists of the latissimus dorsi (lats) and trapezius muscle (traps), along with the glutes, hips, and lower back. Of these muscle groups, the multifidus, transverse abdominis, pelvic floor, and diaphragm muscles are involved in all movement and help to stabilize the spine and pelvis. They are also crucial for maintaining balance.

Strengthening the core will make it easier for you to

stand up from a chair. It will also help you climb stairs.

As you get older, your body starts to lose muscle mass. You can start core exercises at any fitness level. Just remember to listen to your body and avoid activities that could risk your safety. Core exercises can also be helpful for people with back pain. Sitting or lying exercises are good options for those with back problems.

Adding core exercises to your regular workout routine can also help to guard against osteoporosis. The Oxford Textbook of Geriatric Medicine lists falls as the most common cause of fractures in older adults. There are three million emergency room visits each year due to falling injuries. It is essential to prevent these injuries.

Core strengthening exercises for seniors can help prevent injuries. These workouts are safe to do at home and can strengthen the body. They can also reduce lower back pain and chronic pain. When you begin an exercise program, check with a healthcare professional to ensure your condition is compatible with exercising.

If you suffer from arthritis, start slowly, and do not push yourself to the point of pain. You should also focus on the proper execution of the exercise rather than on how many times you do it. Core strengthening exercises can increase balance, stability, and coordination to allow you to continue an independent life. They can also increase your range of motion and help you maintain good posture. Before starting any exercise, make sure you warm up. You should also avoid activity that causes you pain or causes you to feel dizzy. Your core muscles are the foundation of your entire body. The muscles of your spine and hips form a natural girdle around your trunk. A weak core can lead to back strain and other injuries. The core is a collection of muscles located from the ribcage to the pelvis. These muscles support the spine, which in turn keeps you upright.

It is not the first time you have heard that working out the core will improve your posture.

Prevent slouching.

If you are a senior, it is crucial that you keep your

body in shape to prevent slouching. You need to perform core exercises regularly to maintain good posture. Poor posture can affect your vascular system, digestive system, and circulation. This can lead to high blood pressure and varicose veins. Again, as you age, your muscle mass decreases. This is why it is essential to incorporate core strengthening exercises into your weekly workout routine. By strengthening your core, you will increase your overall stability and reduce your risk of injury. These exercises will also help prevent back pain, improve your balance, and make your daily activities easier.

There are three ways that you can perform these core strengthening exercises. They can be performed sitting down, standing up, or lying down. Each of these exercises will target different areas of the midsection. The best part is that you can do them on your own.

One of the significant challenges facing older adults is the development of postural instability. Various factors, including aging, a medical condition, and a lack of muscle strength, can cause this. To combat this, it is essential to work on core exercises that target the midsection and increase balance and coordination. These exercises are also a great way to reduce injury and manage chronic pain. As illustrated in the upcoming chapter, we will cover several core and abdominal exercises to reach your goals. Choosing which exercise works best depends on your needs and fitness level.

ABDOMINALS and OBLIQUES

The Benefits of Strengthening the Abdominals and Obliques

The abdominal muscles and oblique exercises are effective for strengthening your core muscles. The obliques help with side-to-side bending and rotation as part of the core. They also help in protecting the spine from damage. Abdominal muscles and oblique exercises effectively build core strength and provide a stable foundation. In addition to helping prevent lower back strain, the abdominal muscles and obliques help your core perform better in sports, exercises, and everyday functions. The benefits of a strong core are apparent - it supports greater force production. While the Abdominal front muscles are often considered the primary abdominal muscles, the obliques are equally important and need equal attention during abdominal muscle workouts.

Including the obliques in your abdominal muscles workout can improve posture and a thicker core.

Improvements in core stability

A good abdominal muscles and obliques workout is an excellent way to strengthen and stabilize the core. Core stability involves stabilizing the spine and minimizing movements between the vertebrae. It also strengthens the hip and leg muscles. These muscles are often neglected during traditional abdominal muscle routines. Core stability is the ability to do tasks without falling and is an essential component of athletic performance. It can also aid in everyday activities, including standing and walking on two feet. It can also help you maintain a straight posture and be more coordinated as you age. However, despite these benefits, only some scientific studies prove the benefits of abdominal muscles and oblique workouts. A small study in 2011 did not find a significant correlation between core training and functional movements, mainly due to a lack of standardized testing. However, it does show that core strengthening exercises improve posture reaction and movement control.

While an abdominal muscles and oblique workout can improve core stability, a warm-up routine is necessary to prepare the core muscles for a workout. Before you begin any workout, do a few simple cardio exercises to ensure your body is ready to use the core muscles. It is important to remember that abdominal muscles also help stabilize the spine, which is essential for proper form and injury prevention. An abdominal muscles and oblique workout focus on strengthening the side and back muscles, which help with core stability. Training these muscles improves core stability and balance, two of the most important physical functions for a balanced body. It helps your core stay stable and prevent injuries when you fall, so strengthening is essential. When you perform an abdominal muscle and oblique workout, your core muscles should fire before your limbs. The core stability muscles are the foundation of your body, which is why core strength is critical to a healthy running performance. This is particularly true for senior adults who are at risk of falling. Being physically active is one of the best ways to overcome this fear. Getting your abdominal and oblique muscles toned, and limber can help you stay in good shape. They also help you develop a firm waist and prevent back pain.

Pain relief

A good oblique and abdominal muscles workout can help alleviate various pain problems. When these muscles are not used or are weak, they can cause a few issues, particularly in the lower back. A study published in the Journal of Physical Therapy Science showed that patients who included abdominal muscles and oblique exercises in their daily routines reported significantly less chronic back pain. This is good news for those suffering from chronic back pain, which affects more than 50% of the population in the U.S. Abdominal muscles and oblique muscles help maintain proper posture, which helps with movement. This makes them essential for daily life. When strong, the abdominal muscles and obliques support other torso muscles, which can help to breathe.

Training your obliques and abdominal muscles strengthens your entire body. You can also learn to lift heavy weights more quickly if you train your core.

This type of training should be treated with the same intention as the rest of your program. While abdominal muscles and oblique training benefits are apparent, many people neglect these areas. Good abdominal muscles and oblique exercises will help you gain core stability, reduce back pain, and improve flexibility. They can even improve your posture and balance. In addition, regular abdominal muscles and oblique exercises will help your body to lose fat in your midsection and relieve pain in your lower back.

Illustrated Abdominal and Obliques Strengthening Exercises

Seated

Muscle groups activated by the seated abdominal muscles crunch:

- Abdominal muscles and obliques
- Neck

- ◆ Shoulders (anterior, medial, posterior deltoids)
- ◆ Lower Back (latissimus dorsi)
- ◆ Opens the hips.

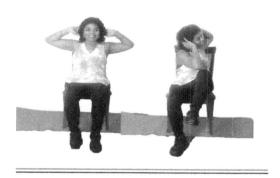

Seated Abdominal Crunches:

Perform Seated, Lying Down, or Standing:

To Begin:

1. Sit leaning slightly backward on a reclining bench or chair with your knees bent at a 90-degree angle.
2. Interlace your fingers behind your head and tighten your abdominal muscles.
3. Lean slightly back so that you graze the chair back. Ensure your core is engaged, hinge your chest forward, and slightly twist to the left, touching your right elbow to your raised left

knee.

4. Return to the starting position and alternate twisting your left elbow towards your right knee.

5. Complete three sets of 5 to 10 reps, increase your reps, sets or both when your strength increases. Wait at least 1-minute in-between sets.

6. If you cannot touch your elbow to your knee, go as far as possible. Your muscles will continue to relax as you continue to perform this exercise.

Muscle groups activated by the seated waist rotation:

◆   Abdominal muscles and obliques
◆   Neck
◆   Shoulders (anterior, medial, posterior deltoids)
◆   Lower Back (latissimus dorsi)
◆   Opens the hips.

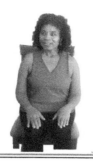 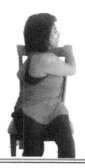

Seated Waist Rotation:

Perform Seated, Standing or Lying Down:

To Begin:

1. Sit straight in your chair and pull in your abdominal muscles while engaging your other core muscles.

2. Rotate at the waist to one side while maintaining a proper upright position.

3. Hold for five seconds and then repeat on the other side.

4. Complete three sets of 5 to 10 reps alternating on each side. Increase your reps, sets or both when your strength increases. Wait at least 1-minute in-between sets.

203

Muscle groups activated by the seated knee tucks:

- ◆ Abdominal muscles and obliques
- ◆ Lower Back (latissimus dorsi)
- ◆ Improves Posture

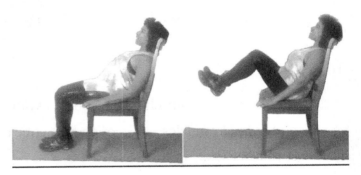

Seated Knee Tucks:

To Begin:

1. Sit up tall on the front half of your chair. Hold on to either side of your chair for added stability.
2. Lean back slightly and engage your abdominal muscles and core.
3. Raise both legs toward your chest, hold for 1-

204

minute, and gradually release.

4. Complete three sets of 5 to 10 reps, increase your reps, sets or both when your strength increases. Wait at least 1-minute in-between sets.

Note: You can also make it a little easier by alternating your legs instead of bringing both legs up simultaneously. You want to use a sturdy, backed chair for this exercise.

Benefits of the seated jumping jacks:

- Cardiovascular Fitness
- Builds Leg Strength
- Total body workout
- Burns Calories
- Increases Bone Density
- Improves Mobility
- Increases Hip Strength
- Improves Coordination

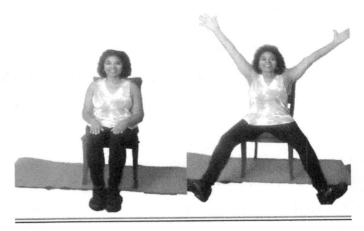

Seated Jumping Jacks:

Perform Seated or Standing:

To Begin:

1. Sit up with your back straight. Place your feet on the floor so they just touch it.

2. Keep your knees close together. Raise your arms overhead while you open your legs out to either side.

3. Repeating this movement in three sets at ten reps can build your endurance and blood flow, which may help you think better. Wait at least 1-minute in-between sets.

Note: Perform your seated jacks quickly to boost cardio and challenge your abdominal and core muscles more. Increase your reps, sets or both when your strength increases.

Standing

Muscle groups activated by the standing dumbbell side bends:

- Obliques and abs (abdominal muscles side wall)
- Shoulders (anterior deltoids)
- Legs (hips)

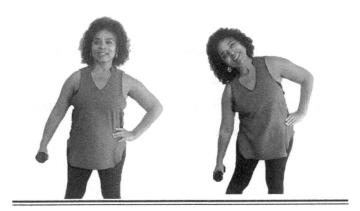

Standing Dumbbell Side Bends:

Perform Standing or Seated:

To Begin:

1. Stand with your feet hip-width apart.
2. Hold a small dumbbell or kettlebell you can safely manage in one hand.
3. Put your free hand on your waist. Bend from your waist toward the side you are holding the weights in.
4. Engage your core to pull your torso back upright.
5. Complete three sets of 5 to 10 reps on one side, then alternate to the other.

208

6 . Increase your weight or sets when your strength increases. Wait at least 1-minute in-between sets.

Note: Use light dumbbells of 1 to 2 pounds initially; you can also use any weighted object, such as canned food items or any small, weighted items.

Pro tip: Ensure you are not sticking your glutes out as you bend.

_____

Muscle groups activated by the standing Overhead Dumbbells Side Bends:

◆ Obliques and abs (abdominal muscles side wall)
◆ Shoulders (anterior, medial deltoids)
◆ Legs (hips)

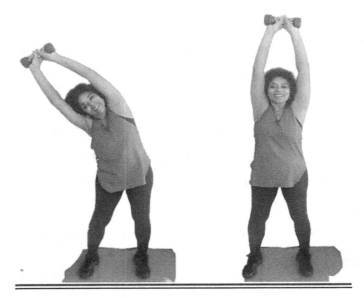

Standing Overhead Dumbbells Side Bends:

Perform Standing or Seated:

To Begin:

1. Stand with your feet hip-width apart.

2. Hold a small dumbbell with both hands.

3. Extend your arms overhead and bend at your waist to the right, keeping your arms straight.

4. Use your core to pull your torso back to the center and repeat on the left side.

5. Complete three sets of 5 to 10 reps alternating

as you go. Increase your weight or sets when your strength increases. Wait at least 1-minute in-between sets.

Note: Use light dumbbells of 1 to 2 pounds initially; you can also use any weighted object, such as canned food items or any small, weighted items.

Muscle groups activated by the woodchop:

◆ Abdominal muscles and obliques
◆ Upper Back
◆ Lower Back (latissimus dorsi)
◆ Shoulders (anterior, medial, posterior deltoids)
◆ Arms (biceps, triceps)
◆ Legs (knees)

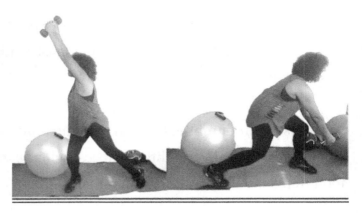

Woodchop:

To Begin:

1. Stand with your feet slightly wider than hip-width apart and hold a small dumbbell with both hands at chest height.

2. Lower the weight to the outside of your left foot, allowing your knees to bend slightly and your feet to pivot.

3. Return the weight across your torso and overhead to the left in a reverse chopping motion.

4. Your feet should pivot in the same direction as the weight.

5. Complete three sets of 5 to 10 reps on

alternating sides. Increase your weight or sets when your strength increases. Wait at least 1-minute in-between sets.

Tip: Make sure you are consciously engaging your core. Increase your speed to create more of a challenge if you can. Use light dumbbells of 1 to 2 pounds initially; you can use any weighted object, such as canned food items or any small, weighted items.

Muscle groups activated by the standing side crunch:

◆   Obliques
◆   Legs (hips)
◆   Abdominal muscles side wall

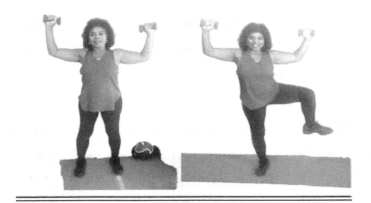

Standing Side Crunch:

To Begin:

1. Stand with your feet slightly wider than hip-width apart.

2. Grab a light dumbbell in each hand and put your arms in a goalpost position.

3. Engage your core; perform a side crunch by bending at your waist and bringing your left leg toward your left elbow.

4. Complete three sets of 5 to 10 reps, alternating as you go.

5. Increase your weight, sets, or both when your strength permits. Wait at least 1-minute in-between sets.

Note: Use light dumbbells of 1 to 2 pounds initially; you can also use any weighted object, such as canned food items or any small, weighted items.

Lying Down

Muscle groups activated by the lying down dumbbell pullover:

- Abdominal muscles and obliques
- Chest (Pectoralis Major and Minor)
- Shoulders (anterior and posterior deltoid)
- Upper Back (trapezius and rhomboids)
- Lower Back (latissimus dorsi)
- Arms (Triceps)

215

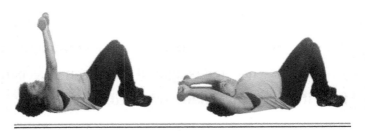

Lying Down Dumbbell Pullover:
Perform Lying Down, Seated or Standing:

To Begin:

1. Lie on your back on the floor and hold two light dumbbells overhead, one in each hand.
2. Press the weight over your chest, then reach back over your head, bending your elbows slightly.
3. Continue until you feel a stretch in your lats, then pull the dumbbell back over your chest.
4. Take a deep breath when you lower the dumbbell behind you.
5. Complete three sets of 5 to 10 reps; increase your weight or sets when your strength increases. Wait at least 1-minute in-between sets.

Note: Use light dumbbells of 1 to 2 pounds initially; you can also use any weighted object, such as canned food items or any small, weighted items.

Muscle groups activated by the crunch:

- ◆ Abdominal muscles and obliques
- ◆ Transverse Abdominis
- ◆ Legs (hips)

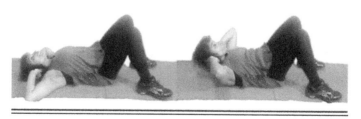

Crunch:

To Begin:

1. Lie on your back, with your knees bent and your feet on a flat surface. Ensure your feet are

shoulder-width apart and pointed straight ahead.

2. Cross your arms on your chest or place your hands behind your ears or head.

3. Slowly crunch your upper body, raising your shoulder blades and keeping your back and lower back stationary. And pause at the top of the move.

4. Slowly lower your upper body back to the starting position.

5. Complete three sets of ten reps, increase your reps, sets or both when your strength increases. Wait at least 1-minute in-between sets.

Muscle groups activated by the toe touches:

◆ Abdominal muscles and obliques
◆ Transverse Abdominis
◆ Legs (hips)

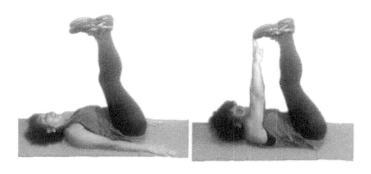

Toe Touches:

To Begin:

1. Lie on your back, with your arms at your sides and legs vertical/straight up in the air.
2. Place your hands together and reach toward your toes, then pause at the top.
3. Slowly lower back down.
4. Complete 5 to 10 reps. Three times, increase your reps, sets or both when your strength increases. Wait at least 1-minute in-between sets.

UPPER BACK

The Benefits of Strengthening the Upper Back

Research has shown that exercise to strengthen the upper back in senior adults reduces the risk of falling. This type of exercise has multiple benefits, including lower limb muscle strengthening and improved balance. However, studies have needed to be more consistent when evaluating specific exercise methods for older adults.

While some researchers have found evidence of effectiveness and safety, others remain unsure of the best method. Regular exercise also helps to strengthen the upper back in senior adults. Weak muscles in the upper back can lead to injuries and damage to the spine. Seniors with weak upper back muscles have an increased risk of falling. They may have difficulty getting up from a chair, which increases the risk of fractures. Seniors who exercise regularly are at lower risk of falling. Regular exercise helps to improve strength and balance, which decreases the risk of falling. Moreover, regular exercise helps to reduce stress on the muscles and joints.

Improves muscle strength.

As a senior, you will want to maintain the muscle strength in your upper back. Practicing them regularly is the key to getting the most out of these exercises. Try to do them three to five times a week. This will improve stamina and help you develop a routine. Strengthening the upper back can help maintain the discs in the spine and keep them functioning correctly. Strengthening the upper back can improve balance and is an excellent way to prevent falls.

Improves flexibility.

Strengthening the upper back for senior adults can benefit physical health and flexibility. Flexibility helps with balance and range of motion. It also reduces the risk of injury. Many health issues can be prevented by exercising, and a solid and flexible upper back can help an older adult remain independent. It is essential to perform upper back strengthening exercises in small sessions as they build stamina. Try to practice at least five exercises three to five days a week. This will build up stamina and familiarity with the routine. Making a back-strengthening routine part of your regular exercise routine will benefit your overall health the most.

Stretching is an essential part of strengthening the upper back. Stretches should be done in a range of motion, and you can do them anywhere. The best time to perform them is immediately after a workout, and it is best to do them when your muscles are warm.

When performing stretches, try to hold each stretch for ten to 20 seconds. During your stretching sessions, include all the major muscle groups, including the upper back and neck. It is also important to stretch the wrists and ankles. Stretching is essential to senior fitness, as it improves flexibility and mobility. It will also help delay the onset of diseases and improve mental health. Moreover, regular physical activity also promotes cognitive and memory function. In addition, stretching exercises will help seniors maintain a strong core and overall balance.

Reduces pain.

Strengthening the upper back can be a vital part of physical therapy, which helps reduce pain and promotes mobility. Choosing balance exercises is essential, incorporating various movements that improve back strength and mobility. When done properly, upper back strengthening exercises can also improve the quality of life and decrease the risk of injury. A lack of back strength has been linked to the development of chronic back pain. By strengthening upper back muscles, seniors can postpone the development of debilitating back pain, hindering their ability to move around and maintain a high quality of life. Before beginning an exercise program, consulting with a physician or other healthcare professional is essential.

Illustrated Upper-Back Strengthening

Exercises

Seated

Muscle groups activated by the seated shoulder shrug:

- ◆ Upper Back (trapezius and rhomboids)
- ◆ Shoulders (anterior and posterior deltoid)
- ◆ Chest (pectoralis major and minor)

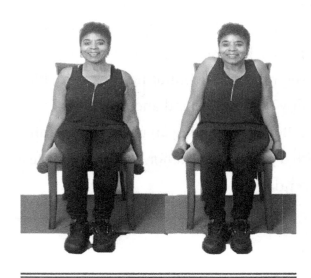

Seated Shoulder Shrug:

Perform Seated or Standing:

To Begin:

1. Sit upright comfortably in a good spinal position, holding a light dumbbell in each hand. Shoulders back and relaxed, looking straight ahead. Slowly raise both shoulders.
2. Hold for 5 seconds, then return to the starting position.
3. Complete three sets of 5 to 10 reps; increase your weight or sets when your strength increases. Wait at least 1-minute in-between sets.

Note: Use light dumbbells of 1 to 2 pounds initially; you can also use any weighted object, such as canned food items or any small, weighted items.

Muscle groups activated by the seated dumbbell shoulder press:

- Upper Back (trapezius and rhomboids)

225

◆ Shoulder (anterior deltoids)
◆ Arms (triceps)
◆ Chest (pectoralis major and minor)

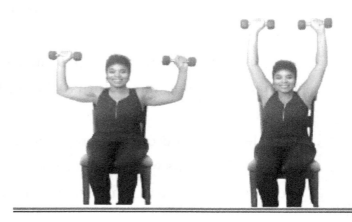

Seated Dumbbell Shoulder Press:
Perform Seated or Standing:

To Begin:

1. Sit with your legs shoulder-width apart and hold a light dumbbell in each hand.
2. With your palms facing forward and your elbows under your wrists, position the dumbbells at your shoulders, with your upper arm parallel to the floor.

3. Push the dumbbells up without fully locking out your elbows.

4. Lower the dumbbells back down to your shoulders and repeat the movement until the set is complete.

5. Complete three sets of 5 to 10 reps; increase your weight or sets when your strength increases. Wait at least 1-minute in-between sets.

Note: Use light dumbbells of 1 to 2 pounds initially; you can also use any weighted object, such as canned food items or any small, weighted items.

Muscle groups activated by the seated lateral dumbbell raise:

◆   Shoulders (medial deltoid)
◆   Upper Back (trapezius and rhomboids)
◆   Arms (triceps)

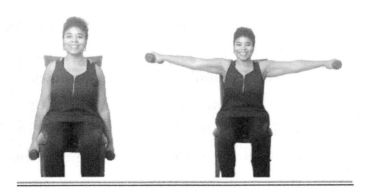

Seated Lateral Dumbbell Raise:

Perform Seated or Standing:

To Begin:

1. Sit with a light dumbbell in each hand at your side, with your palms facing each other. With your back straight and your core activated.
2. Slowly lift both arms out to your side until they are parallel to the floor.
3. Keeping your elbow straight, slowly lower the dumbbells to the starting position and repeat.
4. Complete three sets of 5 to 10 reps, increase your weight or sets when your strength increases. Wait at least 1-minute in-between sets.

Note: Use light dumbbells of 1 to 2 pounds initially; you can also use any weighted object, such as canned food items or any small, weighted items.

Standing

Muscle groups activated by the straight arm pushback:

◆ Upper Back (trapezius and rhomboids)
◆ Shoulders (Rear Deltoids)
◆ Arms (Triceps)

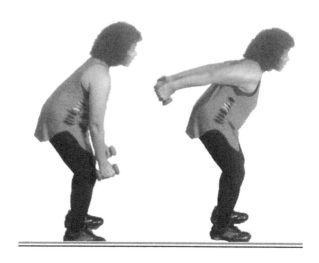

Straight Arm Push Back:

Perform Seated or Standing:

To Begin:

1 . Start with feet, hip distance apart. Engage your abdominals and sit back into a slight squat.
2 . Light dumbbells start at the front of the knees. Keeping the core engaged, press the dumbbells past your hips and return with control. Avoid swinging your arms or bending your elbows.
3 . Complete three sets of 5 to 10 sets
4 . Increase your weight or sets when your strength increases. Wait at least 1-minute in-between sets.

Note: Use light dumbbells of 1 to 2 pounds initially; you can also use any weighted object, such as canned food items or any small, weighted items.

———————————————————

Muscle groups activated by the elbow side extensions.

◆   Upper Back (trapezius and rhomboids)

- ◆ Shoulders (anterior and rear deltoids)
- ◆ Chest (pectoralis major and minor)

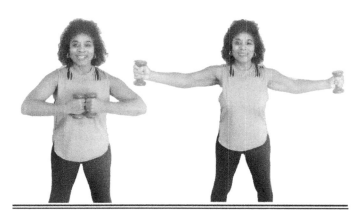

Elbow Side Extensions:
Perform Seated or Standing:

To Begin:

1. Stand with your feet shoulder-width apart, feet flat on the floor. Holding light dumbbells in your hands, elbows bent, palms inward on the chest.
2. Straighten your arms to the sides. Return to the starting position and repeat.

231

3 . Complete three sets of 5 to 10
reps.

4 . Increase your weight or sets when
your strength increases. Wait at
least 1-minute in-between sets.

Note: Use light dumbbells of 1 to 2 pounds initially;
you can also use any weighted object, such as canned
food items or any small, weighted items.

———————————————

**Muscle groups activated by the single-arm
dumbbell rows:**

◆ Upper Back (rhomboids, trapezius)
◆ Shoulders (posterior deltoids)
◆ Arms (biceps)

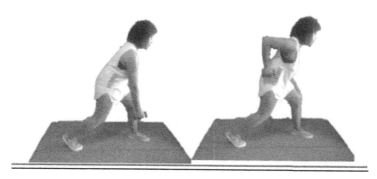

Single Arm Row:

To Begin:

1. Stand in a split stance with your left foot forward with a light dumbbell in your right hand.
2. Slightly hinge over from your hip flexors, keeping your abdominals engaged to protect your low back.
3. Pull the elbow straight past your hip (keep your arms close to the body- do not let your elbow wing out.)
4. Engage and squeeze your back muscles, then lower the dumbbell back to the start position with control.
5. Complete 5 to 10 reps on the right side before

switching to the left side. Complete three sets. Increase your weight or sets when your strength increases. Wait at least 1-minute in-between sets.

Note: Use light dumbbells of 1 to 2 pounds initially; you can also use any weighted object, such as canned food items or any small, weighted items.

Lying Down

Muscle groups activated by the lying down rear deltoids fly:

- Upper Back (trapezius and rhomboids)
- Lower Back (latissimus dorsi)
- Shoulders (rear deltoids)

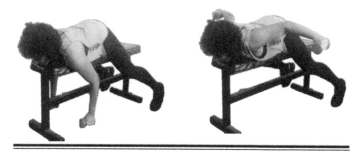

Lying Down Rear Deltoids Fly:

To Begin:

1. Lie on a bench, face down, with a light dumbbell in each hand underneath your shoulders.
2. Slightly bend your elbows and raise your arms to the side until they align with your body.
3. Lower the dumbbells to the floor and repeat.
4. Complete three sets of 5 to 10 reps, increase your weight or sets when your strength increases. Wait at least 1-minute in-between sets.

Note: Use light dumbbells of 1 to 2 pounds initially; you can also use any weighted object, such as canned food or water bottle, or any small, weighted items.

Muscle groups activated by the lying down dumbbell pullover:

◆ Upper Back (trapezius and rhomboids)
◆ Shoulders (Anterior Deltoid)
◆ Abdominal muscles
◆ Chest (Pectoralis Major and Minor)
◆ Lower Back (latissimus dorsi)
◆ Arms (Triceps)

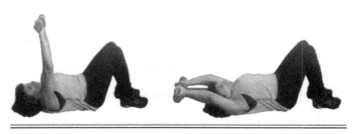

Lying Down Dumbbell Pullover:
Perform Lying Down, Seated or Standing:

To Begin:

1. Lying on your back with your knees up, grasp a light dumbbell, one in each hand, shoulder-width apart.
2. Lift the dumbbells with arms straight as high as you can.
3. With arms extended, lower the dumbbells

straight back with elbows locked without touching the floor.

4. Return to start and repeat.

5. Complete three sets of 5 to 10 reps

6. Increase your weight or sets when your strength increases. Wait at least 1-minute in-between sets.

Note: Use light dumbbells of 1 to 2 pounds initially; you can also use any weighted object, such as canned food items or any small, weighted items.

Muscle groups activated by the walk glute bridge:

- ◆ Lower Back (latissimus dorsi)
- ◆ Legs (glutes, hamstrings, and calves)
- ◆ Abdominal muscles

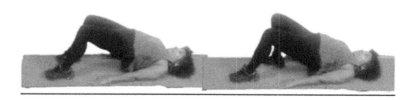

Walk Glute Bridge:

To Begin:

1. Lying on your back with knees bent and feet flat on the floor, hip-width apart.
2. Engage your core, press into your heels, and squeeze the glutes to raise your hips until your body forms a straight line from your knees to the shoulders.
3. Keep hips level and take one step back toward your glutes with the right foot. Do the same with the left foot. Reverse the movement to return to the start.
4. Complete three sets of 5 to 10 step backs on each leg, and increase your reps, sets or both when your strength increases. Wait at least 1-minute in-between sets.

LOWER BACK

The Benefits of Strengthening the Lower Back

Keeping your lower back strong as you age can help prevent arthritic pain. It may also reduce the risk of developing Alzheimer's and other forms of dementia. Exercising the lower back can also help strengthen the isolated lumbar extensor muscles. It is essential to maintain good posture when performing exercises. Chronic low back pain is no fun, but it does not have to be. Fortunately, a lot of hope and healing is out there. A recent study at the Mayo Clinic examined the benefits of exercise to determine if a high-intensity workout can alleviate chronic low back pain symptoms. The results showed that exercise effectively reduces pain and improves overall health. The findings are promising and could make a meaningful contribution to the healthcare debate. As such, researchers are encouraged to glean more information from the study's data sets. Preventing lower back pain by maintaining good posture. Keeping good posture while you work can help prevent lower back pain. Your back is one of the most sensitive parts of your body to injury. This is because your spine is designed to move. A compromised spine can cause muscle strain, fatigue, and joint problems. It can also lead to headaches and breathing problems. Back pain can happen to anyone, and various things can cause it. It can occur gradually, or it can be acute. It can even start in just one area of your back. It can be caused by everyday activities, such as sitting in the same position for long periods. A sudden injury can also cause it. Keeping good posture can help reduce your pain and prevent more serious problems. You may need to change your position and take a break occasionally. This can be as simple as sitting in a chair with good lumbar support or getting up every 30 minutes.

Lower back pain is a common problem for seniors. It can be chronic and can interfere with breathing. Poor body mechanics, overuse, or extra weight often causes it. It can also occur because of spinal degeneration or spinal stenosis. Walking is a great way to strengthen the back and relieve pain. It is also a low-hanging fruit that can reduce back pain, disability, and fear. Walking reduces back pain by improving mobility and quality of life. Performing regular back exercises will reduce pain and help prevent future back problems. Stretching exercises will also strengthen the lower back muscles and help prevent strains and pain in the future. The best exercise for back pain for seniors is walking briskly for at least 20 minutes each day.

Illustrated Lower Back Strengthening Exercises

Seated

Muscle groups activated by the seated cat/cow stretch:

◆ Lower Back (latissimus dorsi)

- ◆ Abdominal muscles
- ◆ Upper Back (trapezius and rhomboids)

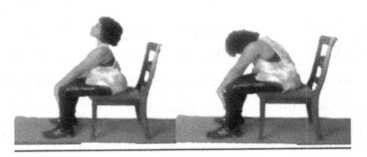

Seated Cat / Cow Stretch:

To Begin:

1. Seat yourself comfortably on a solid chair, with your back straight and unsupported.
2. Keep your feet planted about hip-width apart.
3. Slowly draw your abdominal muscles in, hunching your back and extending your spine.
4. Hold the stretch and the release, pushing your abdominal muscles back outward to the starting position and flexing your spine as you do so.
5. Complete three sets of 3 to 5 stretches or as needed for pain or stiffness. Increase your

number of stretches when your strength increases. Wait at least 1-minute in-between sets.

Muscle groups activated by the seated hip flexor stretch:

◆ Lower Back (latissimus dorsi)
◆ Legs (hips)

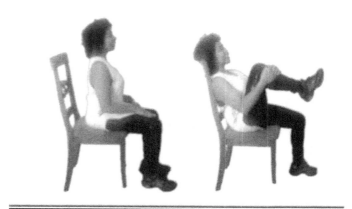

Seated Hip Flexor Stretch:

Perform Seated or Lying Down:

To Begin:

1. Sit toward the front of your chair, place both feet on the floor, and lean back.
2. Hug your right leg into your chest by wrapping your hands around your knee or shin.
3. Keep your back as straight as possible.
4. Repeat on the other side.
5. Hold each side for 30 to 60 seconds.
6. Complete three sets of 30 to 60 seconds. Hold on to each leg alternating.
7. Increase your reps, sets or both when your strength increases. Wait at least 1-minute in-between sets.

Muscle groups activated by the seated forward bend:

- ◆ Lower Back (latissimus dorsi)
- ◆ Legs (glutes, hamstrings, and hips)
- ◆ Spine

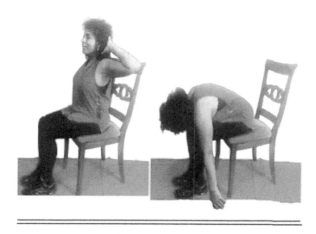

Seated Forward Bend:

To Begin:

1. Sit near the edge of your chair, with your feet firmly on the floor.

2. Slowly lean forward until the chest touches the thighs.

3. Let the head hang down naturally. Allow the arms to hang by your sides. Close your eyes.

4. Breathe calmly and let gravity stretch the back. Feel all the tension in the shoulders goes away. Rest in this posture for 2 minutes.

5. To come up, place the hands on the sides of the seat of the chair, and as you inhale, press down

and lift the torso.

6. Complete three sets of three two-minute poses.
Increase your reps, sets or both when your
strength increases. Wait at least 1-minute in-
between sets.

Standing

Muscle groups activated by the side leg raise:

◆ Lower Back (latissimus dorsi)
◆ Legs (glutes, hips, and hamstrings)

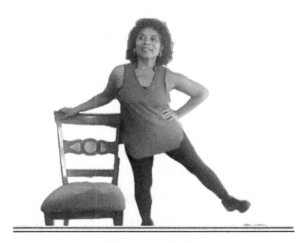

Side Leg Raise:

To Begin:

1. Stand and hold onto a chair for support.
2. Lift one leg to the side, ensuring it is completely aligned from heel to hip.
3. Slowly lower the leg back down, keep your back straight, and maintain a slight bend in the supporting leg. Alternate to the other leg.
4. Complete three sets of 5 to 10 reps, increase your reps, sets or both when your strength increases. Wait at least 1-minute in-between sets.

Muscle groups activated by the reverse standing leg lifts:

- Lower Back (latissimus dorsi)
- Legs (glutes and hamstrings)

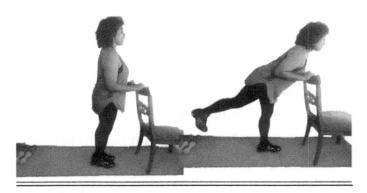

Reverse Standing Leg Lifts:

Perform Standing or Lying Down:

To Begin:

1. Begin by standing straight up, holding onto something sturdy for balance.

2. Engage your core and lift your right foot off the ground slightly, pointing your right leg straight back behind you. Hold for 5 seconds and return your leg underneath you, placing your foot on the floor.

3. Repeat with the left leg, and hold for 5 seconds, making sure to remain steady and keep your core stabilized.

4. Complete three sets of 5 to 10 reps alternating

legs. Increase your reps, sets or both when your strength increases. Wait at least 1-minute in-between sets.

Muscle groups activated by the supported downward dog:

- Lower Back (latissimus dorsi)
- Legs (calves, hamstrings, glutes, and hips)

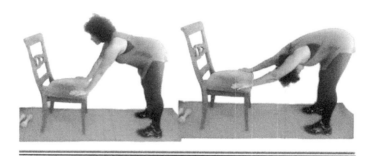

Supported Downward Dog:

To Begin:

1. Stand in front of your chair and place your hands on the seat cushion.

2. Begin to take small steps backward so your

torso can drop down between the chair and your legs.

3 . Walk as far backward as you feel comfortable-- your torso may be parallel to the floor or sloping down at a diagonal. Keep your spine long and straight.

4 . Allow your head and neck to release between your arms. Hold this stretch for 15 to 45 seconds and repeat a few times depending on how tight your back feels; increase your reps, sets, or both when your strength increases. Wait at least 1-minute in-between sets.

Lying Down

Muscle groups activated by the prone straight leg raise:

◆   Lower Back (latissimus dorsi)
◆   Legs (glutes, hamstrings, and quadriceps)

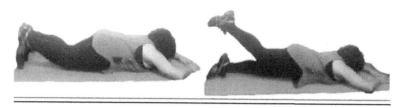

Prone Straight Leg Raises:

Perform Lying Down or Standing:

To Begin:

1. Lie down on your stomach (prone position) and keep your legs stretched out.
2. Tighten the muscles in the hamstring of both legs, lifting one leg toward the ceiling.
3. Hold on to this position for about 5 seconds. Lower your lifted leg, and repeat.
4. Complete 5 to 10 lifts, then switch sides for the other leg. You can add ankle weights as your strength increases. Wait at least 1-minute in-between sets.

Muscle groups activated by the cat/cow pose:

- ◆ Upper Back (trapezius and rhomboids)
- ◆ Lower Back (latissimus dorsi)
- ◆ Shoulders (posterior, medial, anterior deltoids)

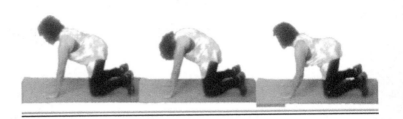

Cat / Cow Pose:

To Begin:

1. Begin comfortably on all fours (weight is on your knees, shins, and hands).

2. Make sure your back and neck are straight but not straining. Relax.

3. Taking a steady inhaling breath, your neck and head gaze upward, and your hips and tailbone mirror in direction. Arch your back in the shape of a "U."

4. When you feel the subtle stretch and your breath is full, you have completed the "cat" pose. Now move on to "cow."

5 . During your exhalation breath, release your head and your bottom down toward the floor. With your hands and knees, gently push onto the floor as your spine arches up in the shape of a rainbow.

6 . In the "cow" pose, you should feel your ab muscles engaged, your lower back stretching, and a slight curve in your neck.

7 . On your next inhale, repeat the cycle. Continue the rhythm, "cat, cow, cat, cow."

8 . Complete three sets of 5 to 10 reps, increase your reps, sets or both when your strength increases. Wait at least 1-minute in-between sets.

Muscle groups activated by the reverse back stretch:

◆ Lower Back (latissimus dorsi)
◆ Legs (hamstrings)
◆ Abdominal muscles

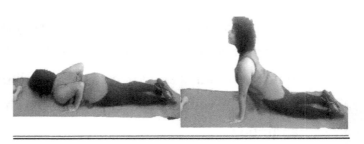

Reverse Back Stretch:

To Begin:

1 . Lie on your stomach with your elbows directly under your shoulders.

2 . Extend your forearms in front with your palms facing down.

3 . Engage your lower back, glutes, and thighs to raise your chest and head.

4 . Gaze straight ahead or slightly up toward the ceiling.

5 . Hold this position for up to 1-minute.

6 . Complete three sets of 5 to 10 reps, increase your reps, sets or both when your strength increases. Wait at least 1-minute in-between sets.

QUADRICEPS

The Benefits of Strengthening the Quadriceps

Whether you are a senior citizen or a child, it is a good idea to exercise the quadriceps muscles to keep you from falling. The quadriceps are the largest muscles in the leg and are essential to your overall health. There are a variety of exercises you can do to improve your fitness and reduce your chances of falling. This section will illustrate quadriceps exercises that will help strengthen them. Increasing the strength of the quadriceps is a great way to keep a senior citizen mobile and pain-free. Strength training can help prevent falls, improve mobility, and decrease the need for medications.

Illustrated Quadriceps Strengthening Exercises

Seated

Muscle groups activated by the heel tap:

◆ Legs (quadriceps, hamstrings, glutes, and hips)
◆ Abdominal muscles

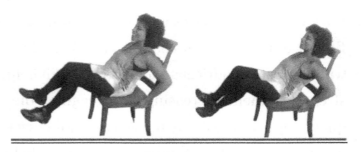

Heel Tap:

Perform Seated or Lying Down:

To Begin:

1. Sit towards the front of your chair, lean back with your lower back straight, contacting the back of the chair.

2. Grasp the rear underside of the chair for support.

3. Lift your legs up so your feet hover one inch off the ground and your thighs are lifting slightly off your chair.

4. Bring your legs 2 to 3 inches apart, then tap your legs together 10 to 15 times.

5. Release and lower your legs.

6. Complete three sets of 5 to 10 reps. Increase your reps, sets or both when your strength increases. Wait at least 1-minute in-between sets.

Muscle groups activated by the crossed leg lift:

◆ Legs (quadriceps, hamstrings, glutes, and hips)
◆ Abdominal muscles

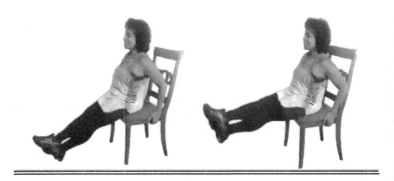

Crossed-Legged Lift:

Perform Seated or Lying Down:

To Begin:

1. Sit near the front of a chair with your back straight and your core engaged. Grip the side of the chair lightly for support.

2. Cross one leg over the other at the ankle. Exhale and extend your bottom leg until it is completely straight and parallel to the ground. (The top leg will lift as well, but keeping it relaxed will allow it to act as a "weight" for the active leg.)

3. Complete three sets of five reps of lifting and lowering, then hold at the top for 10 seconds.

4. Straighten both legs and lower to the ground,

pause, and re-cross with the opposite leg on top. Repeat the exercise with the opposite leg. Increase your reps, sets or both when your strength increases. Wait at least 1-minute in-between sets.

Muscle groups activated by the knee lifts:

◆ Legs (quadriceps, glutes, calves, hamstrings, and hips)

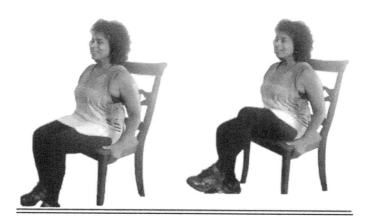

Knee Lifts:

To Begin:

1. Seated in a chair, with your arms resting on your sides with your hands holding the underside of the chair for support, contract your left quadriceps muscles and lift your left leg.
2. Your knee and the back of your thigh should be 2 or 3 inches off the front of the seat.
3. Pause for 3 seconds and slowly lower your leg.
4. Complete three sets of 5 to 10 reps while alternating your legs. Increase your reps, sets or both when your strength increases. Wait at least 1-minute in-between sets.

_____

Standing

Muscle groups activated by the standing mini squat:

◆ Legs (quadriceps and glutes)

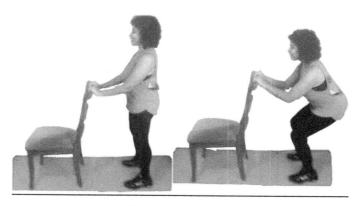

Standing Mini Squats:

To Begin:

1. Stand behind the chair and hold on for support.
2. Bend your knees as far as you comfortably can.
3. Keep your back and head up straight behind your toes.
4. Return to a standing position.
5. Complete three sets of 5 to 10 reps. Increase your reps, sets or both when your strength increases. Wait at least 1-minute in-between sets.

Muscle groups activated by the sit-to-stand:

◆ Legs (quadriceps, glutes, and hamstrings)

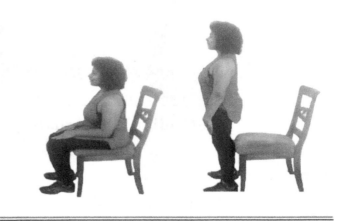

Sit to Stand:

To Begin:

1. Sit toward the front edge of a sturdy chair without armrests. Your knees should be bent, and your feet should be flat on the floor, shoulder-width apart, and underneath your hips.

2. Place your hands lightly on your thigh or each side of the seat. Keep your back and neck straight, with your chest slightly forward.

3. Breathe slowly. Lean forward and slightly shift your weight to the front of your feet.

4. Breathe out as you slowly stand up. Try not to support any weight with your hands.

5. Stand and pause for a full breath in and out.

6. Breathe in as you sit down slowly. Tighten your core and abdominal muscles to control your lowering as much as possible. Slowly lower yourself to the chair, not just drop back into the seat.

7. Breathe out slowly.

8. Complete 5 to 10 times. If needed, complete fewer times until you get stronger. Increase your reps, sets or both when your strength increases. Wait at least 1-minute in-between sets.

Muscle groups activated by the split squat:

◆ Legs (quadriceps and glutes)

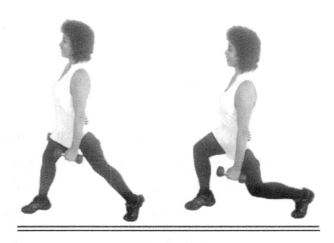

Split Squat:

To Begin:

1. With your feet underneath your shoulders and a light dumbbell in each hand at your sides, step your right foot forward as if you were making a forward lunge, and keep your right heel firmly planted.

2. This is the starting position. (You can also do it with just your body weight to make the exercise easier.)

3. Bend both knees to create 90-degree angles with your legs. Your chest should be upright, and your torso should be slightly forward so

your back is flat and not arched or rounded forward. Your right quad should be parallel to the floor, and your right knee should be above your right foot. Your butt and core should be engaged.

4. Push through your right foot to return to the starting position.

5. Complete three sets of 5 to 10 reps, all on one side at a time, resting at least a minute between sets, then switch sides.

Note: Use light dumbbells of 1 to 2 pounds initially; you can also use any weighted object, such as canned food items or any small, weighted items.

―――――――――――

Lying Down

Muscle groups activated by the prone quad stretch with strap:

◆ Legs (quadriceps, hamstrings, calves, and knees)

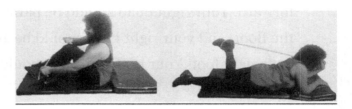

Prone Quad Stretch with Strap:

To Begin:

1. Sit on the floor with your legs extended in front of you, creating an "L" shape.

2. Loop your strap around your right foot. Grasp the strap with your right hand and hold it taut.

3. Roll over onto your stomach while maintaining your grip on the strap.

4. Bend your right knee. Keep your left leg straight.

5. Pull the strap with your hands to bring your right heel closer to your right glute.

6. You should feel a stretch in your right quad. Keep your hips pressed to the floor and slight tension in your abdominal muscles to reduce any tension in your lower back.

7 . Hold the stretch for 30 seconds. Release the tension on the strap.

8 . Complete at least 5 to 10 stretches of 30 seconds each. Repeat this stretch on the left side.

9 . Increase your stretches when your strength increases. Wait at least 1-minute in between stretches.

Muscle groups activated by the side quad stretch.

◆ Legs (quadriceps, hamstrings, calves, and knees)

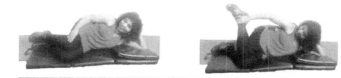

Side Quad Stretch:

To Begin:

1. Lie on your left side, stacking your right leg on top of your left leg and placing your left hand near your left ear to prop up your head.

2. Bend your right leg. Reach your right hand down to grab the top of your right foot.

3. Pull your right foot toward your right glute. Hold for at least 30 seconds.

4. To increase the stretch, make sure your right knee is stacked on top of your left knee. Gently engage your abdominal muscles, tucking your pelvis to increase the stretch further.

5. You should feel this stretch in your right quad.

6. Release the tension.

7. Roll to your right side and repeat this stretch on the left side.

8. Complete three sets of holding for 30 seconds, completing all sets on one leg at a time.

9. Increase your sets when your strength increases. Wait at least 1-minute in between stretches.

———————————————

Muscle groups activated by the prone straight leg raise:

◆ Legs (quadriceps, glutes, and hamstrings)
◆ Lower Back (latissimus dorsi)

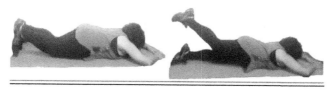

Prone Straight Leg Raises:

Perform Lying Down or Standing:

To Begin:

1. Lie down on your stomach (prone position) and stretch your legs.
2. Tighten the muscles in the hamstring of both legs, lifting one leg toward the ceiling.
3. Hold on to this position for about 5 seconds. Lower your lifted leg, and repeat.
4. Complete 5 to 10 lifts, then switch sides for the other leg. You can add ankle weights as your strength increases. Wait at least 1-minute in-between sets.

HAMSTRINGS

The Benefits of Strengthening the Hamstrings

Developing a routine of hamstring strengthening exercises can help improve strength and stamina. The American Academy of Orthopedics recommends doing a variety of hamstring exercises daily. A hamstring is a group of three muscles at the back of the thigh. They are part of the posterior chain, which helps stabilize the lumbar spine. The hamstrings help with knee flexion and extension. They also help stabilize the hips. The hamstrings play a significant role in shifting load from the knees to the hips. Strong hamstrings will help you maintain good posture and reduce your fall risk. The hamstrings are one of the most important muscle groups in the body. They run from the lower thigh to the base of your glutes. They support your knees and are very important for jumping and walking. They also help to control your hip action during a squat.

Developing muscle growth goals for the hamstrings can help you achieve a balanced body. They are essential for everyday tasks and can help make climbing stairs easier. They can also improve posture and help you to perform better in your sport. If you are new to strength training, you should work the hamstrings once a week, along with your other full-body workout exercises. You can do this alone or integrate it into your lower body warm-up routine. Performing a good amount of hamstring exercises is essential for seniors to maintain their flexibility. Tightness in the hamstrings can cause strain and back pain and limit physical performance. Exercise can improve mobility, muscle quality, and overall performance.

Illustrated Hamstrings Strengthening Exercises

Seated

Muscle groups activated by the seated hamstring stretch:

◆   Legs (hamstrings, knees, and hips)

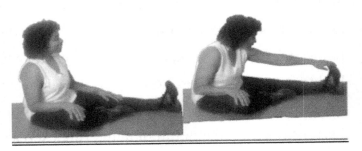

Seated Hamstring Stretch:

To Begin:

1. Select a firm surface to sit on.
2. Next, extend one of your legs out on the surface.
3. Slowly lean forward, breathe, and reach for your thigh, knee, or ankle.
4. Hold this position for 10 to 30 seconds.
5. Repeat with the other side of your body.
6. Complete three sets 5 to 10 times, alternating

on each leg. Increase your reps, sets or both when your strength increases. Wait at least 1-minute in-between sets.

Muscle groups activated by the seated toe touch:

◆ Legs (hamstrings, quadriceps, knees, hips, and glutes)

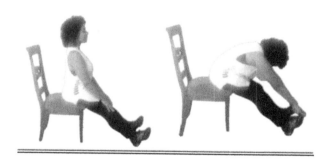

Seated Toe Touch:

Perform Seated or Standing:

To Begin:

1. Sit toward the front of your chair and extend both legs straight with toes flexed back toward

273

your face. If this does not feel good, you can keep your knees bent with your feet flat on the floor.

2. Hinge forward at your hips and allow your torso to fold over your legs as you reach your hands toward your feet. Reach as far as possible, then let your hands rest on your legs or the floor.

3. Allow your neck to release so your head rounds forward. Hold this stretch for 30 to 60 seconds.

4. Complete the stretch for three sets of 5 to 10 times on each leg, alternating. Increase your reps, sets or both when your strength increases. Wait at least 1-minute in-between sets.

Standing

Muscle groups activated by the bending hamstring stretch:

- Legs (hamstrings, glutes, knees, and quadriceps)
- Lower Back (latissimus dorsi)

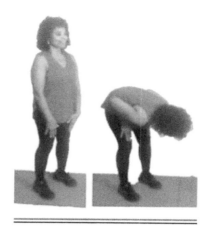

Bending Hamstring Stretch:

Perform Standing or Seated:

To Begin:

1. Stand tall with your arms on your thighs in front of you.
2. Bend forward at the waist until there is a stretch in the hamstring muscle.
3. Hold the stretch for up to 30 seconds.
4. Wait 15 seconds, then repeat three times. Increase your reps when your strength permits.

Muscle groups activated by the single-leg hamstring stretch:

- ◆ Legs (hamstrings, quadriceps, glutes, and knees)
- ◆ Lower Back (latissimus dorsi)

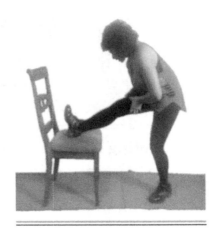

Single Leg Hamstring Stretch:

Perform Standing or Seated:

To Begin:

1. Lay one leg on top of the seat of a chair.
2. Bend forward at the hip, keeping the spine straight.
3. keep the leg on the chair as straight as possible without pain.
4. Hold this stretch for 30 seconds.
5. Complete three sets of 30 seconds hold on

each leg. Aim to perform this exercise twice daily. Increase your sets when your strength increases. Wait at least 1-minute in-between sets.

Muscle groups activated by the Romanian dumbbell deadlift:

◆ Legs (hamstrings, glutes, knees, and quadriceps)
◆ Lower Back (latissimus dorsi)

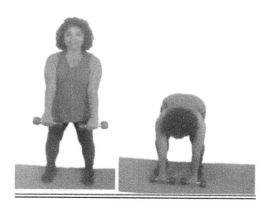

Romanian Dumbbell Deadlift:

To Begin:

1. Standing with feet hip-width apart, knees slightly bent, holding a pair of weights in front of thighs, palms facing your body.
2. Keeping knees slightly bent, press hips back as you hinge at the hips and lower the weights toward the floor.
3. Squeeze your glutes to return to a standing position. That is one rep.
4. Complete three sets of 5 to 10 reps. Increase your weight or set when your strength increases. Wait at least 1-minute in-between sets.

Note: Use light dumbbells of 1 to 2 pounds initially; you can also use any weighted object, such as canned food items or any small, weighted items.

_____

Lying Down

Muscle groups activated by the walk glute bridge:

◆ Legs (glute, hamstrings, and calves)
◆ Abdominal muscles
◆ Lower Back (latissimus dorsi)

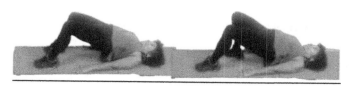

Walk Glute Bridge:

To Begin:

1. Lying on your back with your knees bent and your feet flat on the floor, hip-width apart.
2. Engage your core, then squeeze your glutes to raise the hips until your body forms a straight line from your knees to the shoulders.
3. Keep your hips level and take one step back toward your glutes with the right foot. Do the same with the left. Reverse the movement to return to the start.
4. Complete three sets of 5 to 10 step-backs on each leg. Increase your reps, sets or both when

your strength increases. Wait at least 1-minute in-between sets.

Muscle groups activated by the hip bridge lift:

◆   Legs (hamstrings, quadriceps, and glutes)

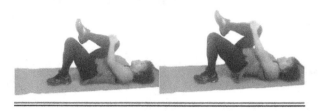

Hip Bridge Lift:

To Begin:
1. Lie on your back with your knees bent and your right leg lifted to your chest.
2. Hug your right leg toward your chest and hold onto that knee.
3. Engage your glutes and lift your hips off the mat.
4. Lower down to the mat. That is one rep.
5. Complete three sets of 5 to 10 reps on one leg

before switching to the other.

6. Increase your reps, sets or both when your strength increases. Wait at least 1-minute in-between sets.

Muscle groups activated by the lying down hamstring stretch:

◆ Legs (hamstrings, knees, quadriceps, glutes, and hips)
◆ Abdominal muscles

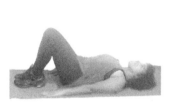 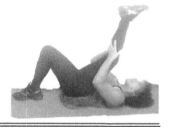

Lying Down Hamstring Stretch:

To Begin:

1. Lie on your back with your knees bent.
2. To stretch the left leg, hold the back of the left

knee with both hands, pull the leg up toward the chest, and slowly straighten the knee until it feels like it is stretching.

3. Hold the stretch for 10–30 seconds.

4. Complete three sets of 10-30 second hold on each leg. Increase your reps, sets or both when your strength increases. Wait at least 1-minute in-between sets.

HIPS

The Benefits of Strengthening the Hips

Whether you are a health professional, a friend, or a relative of a senior citizen, there is no denying the fact that doing regular exercises on the hips can help to stave off the effects of frailty and osteoporosis. It is also suitable for your overall health and improves your mood.

Reduces risk of Alzheimer's disease

Increasing exercise in seniors can help keep them

feeling young and spry. It can also help them maintain their physical fitness and reduce the risk of falls. As a bonus, it can help improve cognitive function and mood. Although the benefits of exercise are well-known, studies have shown that the benefits may be especially beneficial for older adults with dementia. Performing exercises that involve the hips and lower torso will help keep seniors fit and limber. One study found that seniors with dementia are three times more likely to break a hip than those without the disease.

Reduces risk of osteoporosis

Fortunately, there are ways to reduce the risk of osteoporosis when seniors exercise their hips. Osteoporosis is a common disorder that can cause painful broken bones. The condition causes bones to become porous, weakening them and increasing the risk of fractures. The most effective prevention strategies involve a lifetime habit of regular weight-bearing exercise. It has been shown to improve bone density, strengthen bones, and reduce the risk of fractures. Exercise programs for seniors should be tailored to your specific needs. Your doctor should be consulted before you begin any exercise program to ensure your exercise program is safe and effective for you because everyone's situation is different.

Helps retain balance.

Keeping your balance is a crucial component of staying on your feet. This is especially true of older adults, who are more likely to suffer from arthritis and other forms of degenerative joint disease. Often, this condition leads to falls, which can lead to injuries such as broken hips and fractured bones. Regular exercise can help seniors to remain balanced by improving the flexibility and strength of their joints.

Illustrated Hips Strengthening Exercises

Seated

Muscle groups activated by the seated knee raises:

◆ Legs (hips, quadriceps, glutes, calves, and hamstrings)

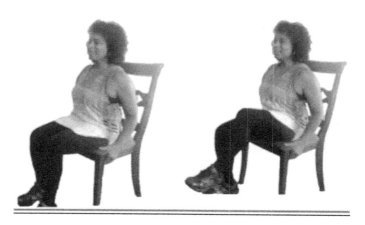

Seated Knee Raises:

Perform Seated or Standing:

To Begin:

1. Seated in a chair, with your arms resting on your sides with your hands holding the underside of the chair for support, contract your left quadriceps muscles and lift your leg.
2. Your knee and the back of your thigh should be 2 or 3 inches off the front of the seat.
3. Pause for 3 seconds and slowly lower your leg.

285

4. Complete three sets of 5 to 10 reps while alternating your legs. Increase your reps, sets or both when your strength increases. Wait at least 1-minute in-between sets.

Muscle groups activated by the seated hip flexor stretch:

◆ Legs (hips)
◆ Lower Back (latissimus dorsi)

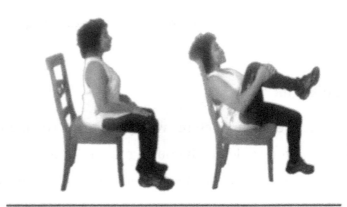

Seated Hip Flexor Stretch:
Perform Seated, Standing or Lying Down:

To Begin:

1. Sit toward the front of your chair, place both feet on the floor, and lean back.
2. Hug your right leg into your chest by wrapping your hands around your knee or shin.
3. Keep your back as straight as possible.
4. Repeat on the other side.
5. Hold each side for 30 to 60 seconds.
6. Complete three sets of 30 to 60 seconds. Hold on to each leg alternating.
7. Increase your reps, sets or both when your strength increases. Wait at least 1-minute in-between sets.

Muscle groups activated by the butterfly pose:

◆ Legs (hips, quadriceps, and knees)
◆ Lower Back (latissimus dorsi)
◆ Groin Area

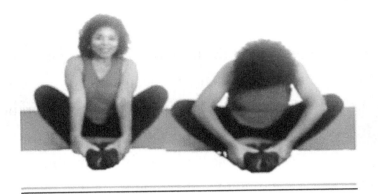

Butterfly Pose:

To Begin:

1 . Sit with your knees bent and the soles of your feet together.

2 . Use your hands to hold the soles of your feet together and your elbows to gently press your knees toward the floor.

3 . Feel an opening in your hips as you release tension.

4 . After 30 seconds, extend your arms in front of you, and come into a forward fold.

5 . Hold this position for up to 1-minute. Complete 3 to 5 sets of holding 1-minute.

6 . Increase your sets when your strength

increases. Wait at least 1-minute in-between sets.

Note: You can deepen the stretch by bringing your heels closer to your body.

Standing

Muscle groups activated by the Frankenstein Walk:

◆ Legs (hips, quadriceps, and hamstrings)

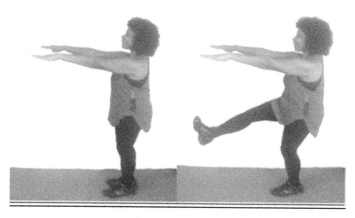

Frankenstein Walk:

To Begin:

1. Stand with your arms extended in front of you, palms facing down.
2. As you move forward, swing your right leg up, with control as far as possible.
3. Lower your right leg to the floor, then swing your left leg up in the same way.
4. Continue for 1-minute, changing direction if your space is limited.
5. Complete three sets of 5 to 10 steps. Increase your steps when your strength increases. Wait at least 1-minute in-between sets.

Note: Consistency will enable you to extend your leg further up.

_____

Muscle groups activated by the step-up:

◆ Legs (quadriceps, hamstrings, glutes, and hips)

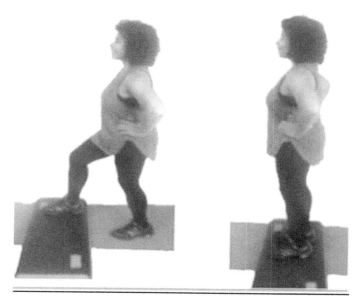

Step Up

To Begin:

1. Place your right foot on a step bench, platform, or the lowest step on a staircase.

2. Keeping your pelvis level, bend your knee and slowly raise your left foot alongside the right foot.

3. Alternate stepping up and down 5 to 10 times.

4. Complete three sets of 5 to 10, Increase your reps, sets or both when your strength increases. Wait at least 1-minute in-between sets.

5. Too easy? Use a higher step or hold a couple of light dumbbells or kettlebells.

Muscle groups activated by the single-leg Romanian deadlift:

- ◆ Legs (hips, hamstrings, and calves)
- ◆ Upper Back (trapezius and rhomboids)
- ◆ Obliques
- ◆ Arms (forearm and wrist)

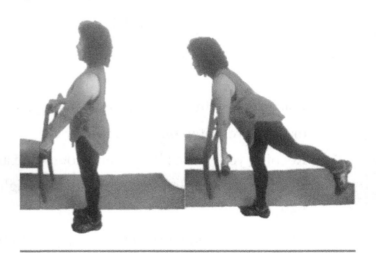

Single-leg Romanian Deadlifts:

To Begin:

1. Stand on your left foot with your knee slightly bent. Hold a light dumbbell in your left hand.
2. Maintain a neutral spine as you hinge to bend toward the floor. Lift your right leg.
3. Come back up to standing. Lower your right leg.
4. Complete three sets of 5–10 reps on each side. Increase your reps, sets or both when your strength increases. Wait at least 1-minute in-between sets.

Note: The goal of the exercise is to lift the free leg parallel to the floor; consistency with this exercise will get you there. Use light dumbbells of 1 to 2 pounds initially; you can also use any weighted object, such as canned food items or small, weighted items.

Lying Down

Muscle groups activated by the knee-to-chest pose:

- ◆ Legs (hips, quadriceps, hamstrings, and knees)
- ◆ Lower Back (latissimus dorsi)

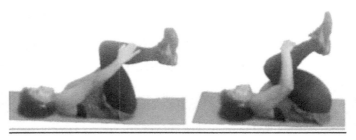

Knee-To-Chest Pose:

To Begin:

1. Lie on your back with your knees bent toward your chest.
2. Wrap your arms around your legs and gently pull your legs into your chest, keeping your lower back stationary and flat against the mat.
3. Hold this position for up to 30 seconds.
4. Complete three sets of this stretch 2–3 times.

294

Increase the number of times when your strength increases. Wait at least 1-minute in-between sets.

Muscle groups activated by the clamshell:

◆ Legs (hips, glutes)
◆ Abdominal muscles
◆ Obliques

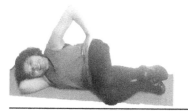 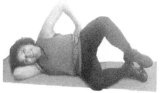

Clam Shell:

To Begin:

1. Lie on your side with bent knees.
2. Rotate your top leg as high as possible, then pause momentarily.
3. Lower to the starting position.

4. Complete three sets of 5–10 reps. Increase your reps, sets or both when your strength increases. Wait at least 1-minute in-between sets.

Muscle groups activated by the donkey kick:

◆ Legs (hips, glutes, knees)

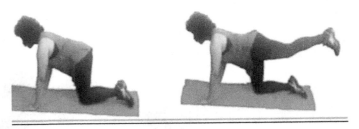

Donkey Kick:

To Begin:

1. While on your hands and knees, lift your left knee, keeping it bent as you kick outward.
2. Push the bottom of your foot out away from you.
3. Return to the starting position.

4. Complete three sets of 5 to 10 kicks alternating legs. Increase your sets when your strength increases. Wait at least 1-minute in-between sets.

GLUTES

The Benefits of Strengthening the Glutes

Caring for our glutes is a great way to maintain our muscles and bones and prevent falls and injuries. It also helps to strengthen the lower body and improve our balance.

Older adults have different physical limits. This means they need to be cautious when exercising. For example, if you are a senior with arthritis, you may not be able to perform the same exercise routine as someone who does not have arthritis. In these cases, you should start with a smaller, more gradual level of exercise. However, you should always seek medical advice before starting a new exercise program. You can find out what exercises are appropriate for your body and what activities you should avoid.

Increasing physical activity can reduce the symptoms of anxiety and depression. It also has decreased the risk of heart disease and colon cancer. Regular exercise also reduces the risk of high blood pressure and insomnia.

Prevent falls.

Exercising your glutes can reduce your chances of falling. They are a vital part of the body's braking mechanism; their job is to abduct and rotate the hips. It is an excellent idea to do some exercises that work the glutes, and you should also stretch them after you finish exercising them. A good rule of thumb is to start with small reps and gradually increase them over a few weeks. This will allow you to work your glutes without damaging your body.

Strengthen legs and glutes.

Performing exercises designed to strengthen your legs and glutes can help protect your joints from injury and keep you active for longer. This is a good thing if you are older. Moving can also help keep your bones and joints healthy and provide several other benefits. Performing strength training exercises can also help manage hip and knee problems. The key is to be consistent with your exercise routine.

Illustrated Glutes Strengthening Exercises

Seated

Muscle groups activated by the chair side lunge:

◆   Legs (glutes, quadriceps, hamstrings, and calves)
◆   Abdominal muscles
◆   Obliques

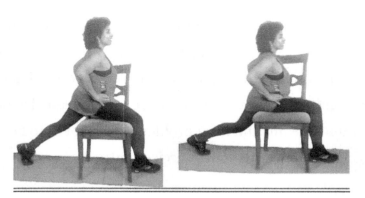

Chair Side Lunge:

To Begin:

1. Begin by straddling and hovering above a chair without an armrest and maintaining proper alignment with your head, shoulders, and hips.

2. Lower your body without resting on the chair to feel the stretch in the front of the hip.

3. Hold this position for 10 seconds. Relax and repeat the movement on the opposite side.

4. Complete three sets of 10 seconds and hold on each leg separately. Increase your hold time or sets when your strength increases. Wait at least 1-minute in-between sets.

Muscle groups activated by the sit-to-stand:

◆   Legs (glutes, hips, quadriceps, and hamstrings)

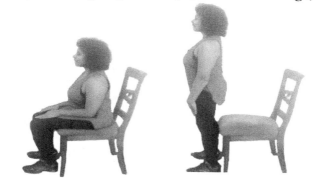

Sit to Stand:

To Begin:

1. Sit towards the front edge of a sturdy chair without an armrest.

2. Your knees should be bent, and your feet should be flat on the floor and shoulder-width apart and underneath your hips.

3. Place your hand lightly on your thigh or each side of the seat.

4. Keep your back and neck straight, with your

chest slightly forward.

5. Breathe slowly, lean forward, and slightly shift your weight to the front of your feet.

6. Breathe out as you slowly stand up. Try not to support any weight with your hands.

7. Stand and pause for a full breath in and out.

8. Breathe in as you sit down slowly. Tighten your core and abdominal muscles to control your lowering as much as possible. Slowly lower yourself to the chair, not just drop back into the seat.

9. Breathe out slowly.

10. Complete three sets of 5 to 10 reps. Increase your reps, sets or both when your strength increases. Wait at least 1-minute in-between sets.

_____

Muscle groups activated by the Side Chair Cross Leg Lift:

◆ Legs (glutes, hips, and quadriceps)
◆ Abdominal muscles

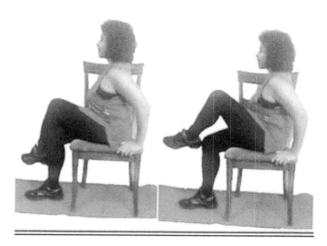

Side Chair Cross Leg Lift:

To Begin:

1. Sit on your right side in a chair and sit sideways with the left leg on top of the right leg.
2. Raise your left leg like opening a clam shell.
3. Lower your left leg without resting it on top of the right leg and repeat.
4. Complete three sets of 5 to 10 reps and repeat on the other leg. Increase your reps, sets or both when your strength increases. Wait at least 1-minute in-between sets.

Standing

Muscle groups activated by the standing mini squats:

- ◆ Legs (glutes, quadriceps, knees, and hamstrings)
- ◆ Abdominal muscles

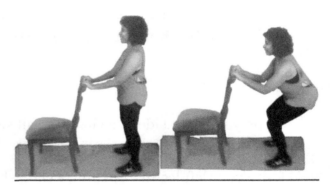

Standing Mini Squats:

To Begin:

1. Stand behind the chair and hold on for support.
2. Bend your knees as far as you comfortably can.

3. Keep your back and head up straight behind your toes.

4. Return to a standing position.

5. Complete three sets of 5 to 10 reps. Increase your sets or reps when your strength increases. Wait at least 1-minute in-between sets.

Muscle groups activated by the lunge:

◆ Legs (glutes, hips, hamstrings, quadriceps, calves, and knees)

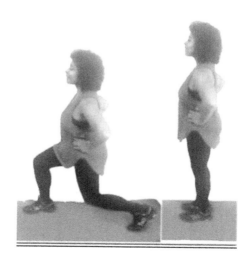

Lunge:

To Begin:

1. From a standing position, look straight ahead and take a generous step forward with your right foot.
2. Keep your trunk upright throughout the movement.
3. Bend your extended knee and transfer your weight onto your right leg. Slowly lower yourself into the lunge until your left knee hovers above or softly touch the floor.
4. Your right knee should be directly above your right ankle.
5. Step back into a standing position.
6. Repeat with your left leg in front.
7. Complete three sets of 5 to 10 lunges alternating legs. Increase your reps, sets or both when your strength increases. Wait at least 1-minute in-between sets.

_____

Muscle groups activated by the step-up:

◆ Legs (quadriceps, hamstrings, glutes, hips, and knees)

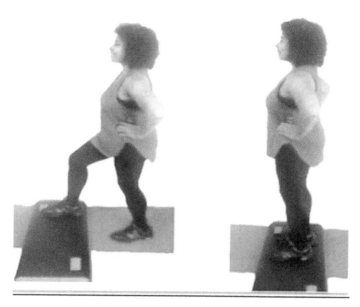

Step Up:

To Begin:

1. Place your right foot on a step bench, platform, or the lowest step on a staircase.
2. Keeping your pelvis level, bend your knee and slowly raise your left foot alongside the right

307

foot.

3. Alternate stepping up and down 5 to 10 times.

4. Complete three sets of 5 to 10 up and down steps per leg, resting at least 1-minute between sets.

5. You can make it more of a challenge by using a higher step or holding a couple of small dumbbells (1 to 2 pounds) or kettlebells.

Lying Down

Muscle groups activated by the glute bridge:

◆ Legs (glutes, hamstrings, and knees)
◆ Abdominal muscles

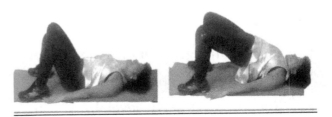

Glute Bridge:

To Begin:

1. Start by laying on your back on a comfortably padded floor, such as a carpet or yoga mat. Bring the soles of your feet to the floor with your knees pointing up to the ceiling. Your arms are on the floor, along the sides of your body, shoulders dropped away from the ears.

2. Engaging your outer hips and butt, push your hips up to raise off the floor slightly. Raise your hips and pelvis as high as you can off the floor. You may feel your core engage.

3. Gently lower your hips back down to the floor. Release your muscles and relax.

4. Complete three sets of 5 to 10 reps, increase your reps, sets or both when your strength increases. Wait at least 1-minute in-between sets.

Muscle groups activated by the clamshell:

- Legs (hips, glutes)
- Abdominal muscles
- Obliques

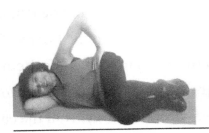 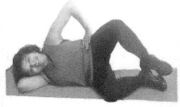

Clam Shell:

To Begin:

1. Lie on your side with bent knees.
2. Rotate your top leg as high as possible, then pause momentarily.
3. Lower to the starting position.
4. Complete three sets of 5 to 10 reps. Increase your reps, sets or both when your strength increases. Wait at least 1-minute in-between sets.

Muscle groups activated by the donkey kick:

◆   Legs (glutes, hips, and knees)

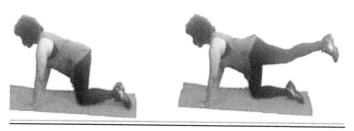

Donkey Kicks:

To Begin:

1. While on your hands and knees, lift your left knee, keeping it bent as you kick outward.
2. Push the bottom of your foot out away from you.
3. Return to the starting position.
4. Complete three sets of 5 to 10 kicks alternating legs. Increase your kicks when your strength increases. Wait at least 1-minute in-between sets.

KNEES

The Benefits of Strengthening the Knees

Keeping your knees strong is very important, especially as a senior. Fortunately, there are many exercises you can do to help you maintain healthy knees. Some exercises you can do include walking, running, climbing, squatting, and strength training which are covered in this book. You can do these exercises at home or join a gym. Whatever you decide, make sure you are doing them correctly.

Managing arthritis

Symptoms of arthritis include pain, stiffness, and inflammation. This can affect a person's quality of life and limit their ability to perform daily tasks. This condition can lead to disability and disability-related healthcare costs. Managing arthritis can help seniors remain active and comfortable. Arthritis is the most common musculoskeletal condition in older adults.

312

The most common form of arthritis is osteoarthritis. In osteoarthritis, the cartilage in the joints breaks down. Research has found that seniors are at high risk for knee osteoarthritis. When seniors have osteoarthritis, they are at risk for knee pain, stiffness, and joint swelling. Pain-relieving injections and physical therapy can help seniors to manage arthritis and remain mobile. Research has shown that exercise may decrease the pain and disability of arthritis. Exercise reduces pain, improves mobility, and improves muscle tone.

Balance problems

Getting older means you will have to cope with various health issues. A number of these issues may increase your chances of falling. However, there are some things you can do to keep yourself afloat. Among these are a variety of strength and flexibility exercises. These can include walking heel to toe and even leg lifts while seated. Another apropos way to maintain your balance is to exercise the knees.

Illustrated Knees Strengthening Exercises

Seated

Muscle groups activated by the seated knee extension:

◆ Legs (knees and quadriceps)

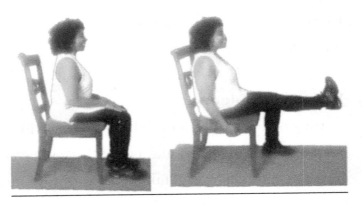

Seated Knee Extension:

Perform Seated, Standing or Lying Down:

To Begin:

1. Sit on the edge of your chair with your hands gripping the side for extra support if needed.

2 . Keep both feet flat on the floor with your knees bent.

3 . Straighten your right leg until it is parallel to the floor, squeezing your quads at the top.

4 . Return the leg to the ground and repeat with the other leg.

5 . Complete three sets of 5 to 10 reps, alternating legs.

6 . Increase your reps, sets or both when your strength increases. Wait at least 1-minute in-between sets.

Muscle groups activated by the hamstring drag:

◆   Legs (knees, hamstrings, and calves)

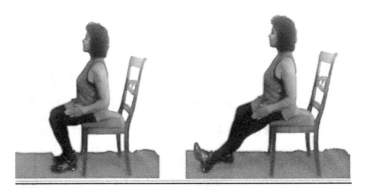

Hamstring Drag:

To Begin:

1. Begin in an upright sitting position at the front of your chair, with your legs shoulder-width apart and maintaining proper alignment with your head, shoulders, and hips.

2. Place your hands just above your knees and straighten one leg in front of your body.

3. Engage your core, then drag your heel back along the floor slowly.

4. Return to the starting position and repeat the movement on the opposite side.

5. Complete three sets of 5 to 10 reps alternating legs. Increase your sets when your strength increases. Wait at least 1-minute in-between sets.

Muscle groups activated by the chair side lunge:

- Legs (knees, glutes, quadriceps, hamstrings, and calves)
- Abdominal muscles
- Obliques

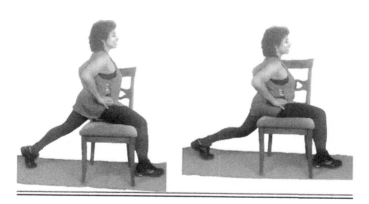

Chair Side Lunge:

To Begin:

1. Begin by straddling and hovering above a chair without an armrest and maintaining proper

alignment with your head, shoulders, and hips.

2. Lower your body without resting on the chair to feel the stretch in the front of the hip.

3. Hold this position for 10 seconds. Relax and repeat the movement on the opposite side.

4. Complete three sets of 10 seconds and hold on each leg separately. Increase your reps, sets or both when your strength increases. Wait at least 1-minute in-between sets.

Standing

Muscle groups activated by the standing mini squats:

- Legs (knees, glutes, quadriceps, and hamstrings)
- Abdominal muscles

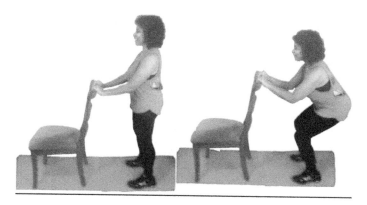

Standing Mini Squats:

To Begin:

1. Stand behind the chair and hold on for support.
2. Bend your knees as far as you comfortably can.
3. Keep your back and head up straight behind your toes.
4. Return to a standing position.
5. Complete three sets, 5 to 10 reps, increase your reps, sets, or both when your strength increases. Wait at least 1-minute in-between sets.

319

Muscle groups activated by the knee flexion:

◆   Legs (knees and hamstrings)

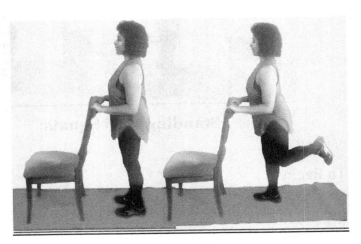

Knee Flexion:

Perform Standing, Seated, or Lying Down:

To Begin:

1. Stand behind a chair using the back of the chair for balance.
2. Flex your left leg to about a ninety-degree angle, hold for ten seconds, then return to the starting position.
3. Switch legs and do ten reps with each leg.

320

4. Complete three sets of ten reps alternating legs.

5. Increase your reps, sets, or both when your strength increases. Wait at least 1-minute in-between sets.

Muscle groups activated by the step-up:

◆ Legs (knees, quadriceps, hamstrings, glutes, and hips)

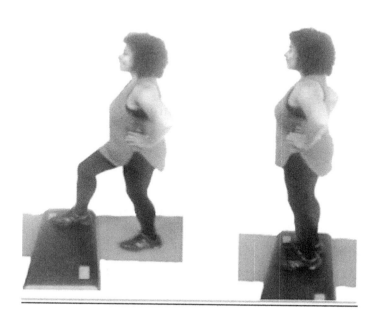

Step Up:

To Begin:

1. Place your right foot on a step bench, platform, or the lowest step on a staircase.
2. Keeping your pelvis level, bend your knee and slowly raise your left foot alongside the right foot.
3. Alternate stepping up and down 5 to 10 times.
4. Complete three sets of 5 to 10 up and down steps per leg; increase your sets when your strength increases, resting at least 1-minute between sets.
5. You can make it more of a challenge by using a higher step or holding a couple of small dumbbells (1 to 2 pounds) or kettlebells.

Lying Down

Muscle groups activated by the donkey kick:

◆ Legs (knees, hips, and glutes)

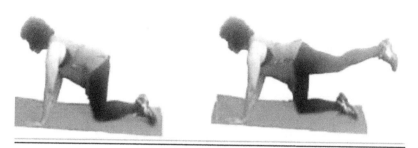

Donkey Kicks:

To Begin:

1. While on your hands and knees, lift your left knee, keeping it bent as you kick outward.
2. Push the bottom of your foot out away from you.
3. Return to the starting position.
4. Complete three sets of 5 to 10 kicks alternating legs. Increase your kicks when your strength increases. Wait at least 1-minute in-between sets.

Muscle groups activated by the straight leg raises with knee bend:

◆   Legs (knees, quadriceps, and hips)

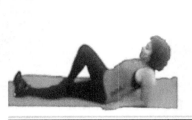 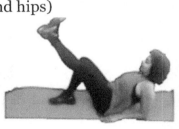

Straight Leg Raise with Knee Bend:

To Begin:

1. Lie on your back on the floor or another flat surface.

2. Bend one knee and place your foot flat on the floor.

3. Keeping the other leg straight, raise it to the height of the opposite knee.

4. Complete three sets of 5 to 10 reps, then alternate legs.

5. Increase your reps, sets, or both when your strength increases. Wait at least 1-minute in-between sets.

Muscle groups activated by the prone straight leg raise:

◆ Legs (knees, quadriceps, back, glutes, and hamstrings)

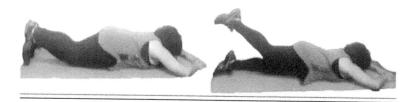

Prone Straight Leg Raises:
Perform Lying Down or Standing:

To Begin:

1. Lie down on your stomach (prone position) and stretch your legs.
2. Tighten the muscles in the hamstring of both legs, lifting one leg toward the ceiling.

3. Hold on to this position for about 5 seconds. Lower your lifted leg, and repeat.

4. Complete 5 to 10 lifts, then switch sides for the other leg. You can add ankle weights as your strength increases or increase the number of lifts. Wait at least 1-minute in-between sets.

CALVES

The Benefits of Strengthening the Calves

The muscles in your calf include the gastrocnemius and the soleus. These muscles work together to form the Achilles tendon, which helps to push your heel off the ground. Strong calves are the foundation for stability in our body while we stand, jump, or run. By strength-training your calves, you will improve your foot, ankle, and knee stability, improving your balance and enabling you to decelerate more effectively. Keeping the leg muscles strong is essential, as this helps to avoid circulation problems. One way to do this is to exercise the calf muscles.

Improved Performance
The calves are a significant muscle group for running, jumping, and other fast-moving activities. They are responsible for generating power during these activities, so muscular calves can help you improve your performance

and increase your explosiveness. The larger of the two calf muscles, the gastrocnemius, starts at the bottom of your thigh bone and attaches to your Achilles tendon. Exercising the calf muscles can also provide relief from conditions like plantar fasciitis and Achilles tendonitis. You can target these muscles by performing various exercises, including calf raises, which are simple and effective. Several 3-5 methodical reps are enough to build calf base strength.

Increased Stamina

Stamina is a critical fitness component, and it helps you perform various types of physical activities for long periods. It can be achieved through diet, exercise, and a healthy lifestyle.

Strengthening the calves is one of the best ways to improve your stamina. Strengthening the calf muscles can help you walk with more confidence and stability.

/ SENIOR STRENGTH EXERCISES 60+

Another way to increase your stamina is by swimming. Regular swimming workouts help increase your endurance by providing oxygen to your lungs and building up your cardiovascular system.

Increased Flexibility

A strong and flexible calf is a crucial part of any athletic performance. It provides critical stabilization during walking, running, and jumping, explains Jason Loebig, Nike training and running coach. Strengthening the calves can reduce the risk of nagging injuries, such as shin splints and Achilles tendonitis, says Cody Braun, NASM-certified personal trainer. It also helps prevent chronic conditions like plantar fasciitis and heel pain.

During weight-bearing exercises, such as squats and lunges, tight calf muscles can limit ankle mobility, making it difficult to perform all required movements.

To increase flexibility, try a variety of calf stretches and exercises. These can be performed either before or after a leg-intensive workout.

Illustrated Calves Strengthening Exercises

Seated

Muscle groups activated by the seated calf raises:

◆   Legs (calves)

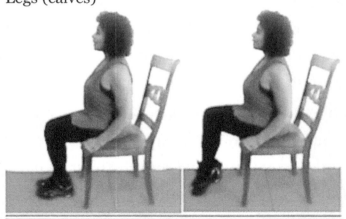

Seated Calf Raise:

Perform Seated or Standing:

To Begin:

1. Sitting up tall in your chair, your feet hip-width apart.
2. Bring your feet back so your heels are behind your knees.
3. From this position, lift your heels off the floor, coming up onto your toes.
4. Hold briefly and gently lower your heels back down.
5. Complete three sets of 10 to 15 reps. Once strength increases, a small weight can be placed on the knees. Increasing your sets or reps is another option, or you can do both. Wait at least 1-minute in-between sets.

Standing

Muscle groups activated by the standing

forward bend pose:

- ◆ Legs (calves, hamstrings, and glutes)
- ◆ Spine Muscles

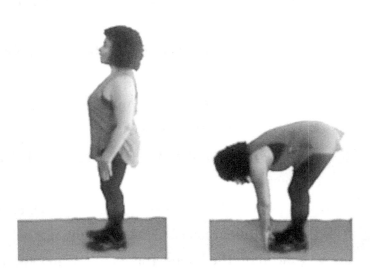

Standing Forward Bends Pose:

Perform Standing or Lying Down:

To Begin:

This pose releases tension in your head, neck, and back. You will also loosen up your spine and legs. To deepen this stretch, bend your knees and place your palms facing upward underneath your feet.

1. Stand with your feet hip-distance apart or slightly wider.
2. Hinge at your hips to lower your torso toward your legs.
3. Bend your knees to a comfortable degree.
4. Place your hands on your legs, a block, or the floor.
5. Draw your chin toward your chest and let your head hang heavily.
6. Complete three sets of forward bends, waiting for at least 1-minute between sets.

Muscle groups activated by the calf stretch:

◆ Legs (calves, knees, and quadriceps)

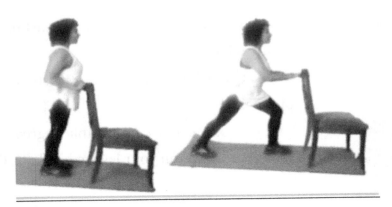

Calf stretches:

To Begin:

1. Place your hands on the back of the chair for support.
2. Step back with your right foot while pointing both feet towards the chair.
3. Lean forward and keep your right heel on the floor.
4. Hold for 30 seconds.
5. Complete three sets of 5 to 10 reps alternating legs.
6. Increase your reps, sets, or both when your strength increases. Wait at least 1-minute in-between sets.

Muscle groups activated by the standing calf raises:

◆ Legs (calves, ankle and feet, hamstring, and quadriceps)

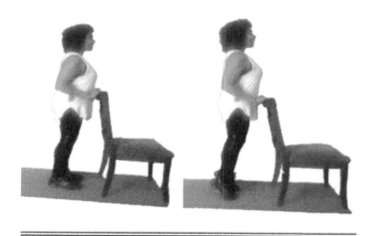

Standing Calf Raises:

Perform Standing or Seated:

To Begin:

1. Stand straight with your feet hip-width apart, arms holding the back of the chair for support.

2. Keeping your back straight, slowly rise on the toes of both feet, raising your heels as high as you can.

3. Pause at the top, then slowly lower your heels.

4. Complete three sets, 5 to 10 reps per set. Increase your reps, sets, or both when your strength increases. Wait at least 1-minute in-between sets.

Lying Down

Muscle groups activated by the glute bridge:

◆ Legs (calves, glutes, hamstrings, and knees)
◆ Abdominal muscles

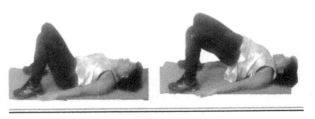

Glute Bridge:

To Begin:

1. Start by laying on your back on a comfortably padded floor, such as a carpet or yoga mat. Bring the soles of your feet to the floor with your knees pointing up to the ceiling. Your arms are on the floor, along the sides of your body, shoulders dropped away from the ears.

2. Engaging your outer hips and butt, push your hips up to raise off the floor slightly. Raise your hips and pelvis as high as you can off the floor. You may feel your core engage.

3. Gently lower your hips back down to the floor. Release your muscles and relax.

4. Complete three sets of 5 to 10 reps; increase your reps, sets, or both when your strength increases. Wait at least 1-minute in-between sets.

———————————————————

ANKLES and FEET

The Benefits of Strengthening the Ankles and Feet

Performing a routine of foot and ankle exercises is one of the best things you can do to keep your feet and ankles strong. Performing stretching routines and strengthening your feet and ankles can help prevent falls and relieve pain. Increasing intrinsic foot muscle strength can improve balance and reduce the risk of falls in older adults. In addition, strengthening these muscles may prevent the onset of foot problems such as plantar fasciitis. Having a good exercise routine can be very beneficial to the health of your ankles and feet. During any movement, the ankle and feet are the first contact points for force transmission. This makes the feet a vital joint, and exercising them is a great way to improve your overall health. Keeping your feet and ankles in tip-top shape will help to prevent aches, pains, and injuries. The right foot and ankle exercises can help to improve posture, strengthen core muscles, and even improve balance. They can also help to prevent future injuries. However, if you are recovering from an injury, it is a good idea to avoid weight-bearing activities. This is particularly true if you are overweight. A high-impact workout can overload your ankles and feet and put you at risk for strains and sprains. This is why it is a good idea to participate in a low-impact workout while you are recuperating.

The feet and ankles can be the source of many energy leaks if it is not properly functioning. The brain is responsible for proprioception, or the ability to identify your body position in space. A good foot and ankle workout will improve your proprioception, and a proper warm-up is the best start. There are many foot and ankle exercises to choose from. Some of which are illustrated in these pages. The best way to select the correct exercises for your fitness level is to talk to your healthcare provider about the best options. The foot and ankle have a lot of muscles and tendons, and they need to be adequately trained to function correctly. The most essential part of any exercise is ensuring you perform it safely. While the

foot and ankle have many functions, the most
important is strength.

Illustrated Ankles and Feet Strengthening Exercises

Seated

Muscle groups activated by the ankle and foot circles:

◆   Legs (ankle, foot, and calves)

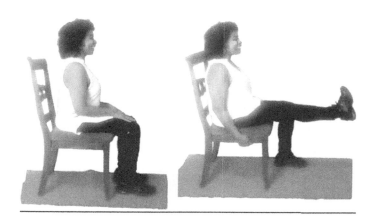

Seated Ankle and Foot Circles:

Perform Seated, Standing, or Lying Down:

To Begin:

1. Sit tall in a chair or a bench, with your hands gripping the side of the chair for extra balance.
2. Extend your right leg as far as possible while keeping your left foot on the floor.
3. Point your toe up and then rotate your foot once clockwise.
4. Rotate the same foot counterclockwise.
5. Complete three sets of 5 to 10 reps, alternating your feet. Increase your reps, sets, or both when your strength permits. Wait at least 1-minute in-between sets.

Toe Raises:

To Begin:

1. Start seated with your feet flat on the floor. Rest your hands on your lap or the sides of your chair.
2. Lift your toes on your right foot, keeping the left foot planted firmly on the floor.
3. Hold for 3 to 5 seconds.
4. Lower your toes.
5. Complete three sets of 10 to 15 times on each foot. Increase your reps, sets, or both when your strength permits. Wait at least 1-minute in-between sets.

Towel Toe Curls

Sit in a sturdy chair, place your foot on a towel on the floor, and scrunch the towel toward you with your toes.

Then, also using your toes, push the towel away from you.

Make this exercise more challenging by placing a weighted object on the other end of the towel, such as a can of any food item.

Complete three sets of 5 to 10 back-and-forth movements, depending on your strength level. Wait at least 1-minute in between sets.

———————————

Toe Splay:

To Begin:

1. Sit in a straight-backed chair with your feet gently resting on the floor.
2. Spread all your toes apart as far as comfortable.
3. Hold for five seconds.
4. Complete three sets of ten times on each foot. Increase your reps, sets, or both when your strength permits. Wait at least 1-minute in-between sets.

Note: You can make this exercise more challenging by

looping a rubber band around the toes of each foot.

Standing

Muscle groups activated by the high marching:

◆   Legs (ankle, feet, quadriceps, hamstrings, and knees)

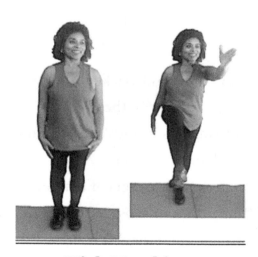

High Marching:

To Begin:

1. Stand facing forward with your feet together and arms at your sides.
2. Raise one knee as high as comfortable and then lower it down. As you mention the knee, shift your weight onto the other leg.
3. Repeat on the other side as if you were marching.
4. Complete three sets of 5 to 10 alternating legs. Increase your reps, sets, or both when your strength permits. Wait at least 1-minute in-between sets.

Muscle groups activated by the single leg raise:

◆   Legs (ankle, feet, knees, hamstrings, and quadriceps)

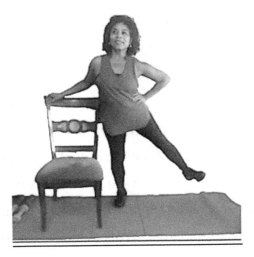

Single Leg Raise:

To Begin:

For this exercise, set up near something you can hold on to, such as a chair, table, or kitchen worktop. As your balance improves, you can do this exercise without assistance.

1. Stand with your feet hip-width apart, arms by your sides, looking straight forward.

2. Soften your left knee and lift your foot so it is entirely off the ground, so you are balancing your weight on your right leg. Make sure to hold your weight straight over your ankles.

3. Complete three sets of 5 to 10 reps holding your

foot ankle high for 10 seconds. Alternate to the other legs. Increase your reps, sets, or both when your strength permits. Wait at least 1-minute in-between sets.

Muscle groups activated by the ankle circles:

◆ Legs (ankles and feet plus calves)

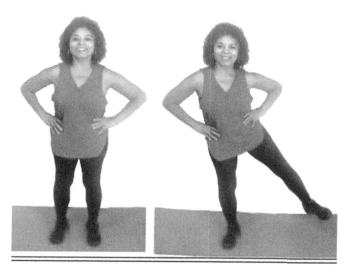

Standing ankle Circles:

Perform Standing, Seated, or Lying Down:

To Begin:

1. Stand tall with your abdominals engaged and your hands on your hips or by your side.
2. Shift your weight to your right leg and balance on your right leg and raise your left leg and rotate your ankles in a circular motion, clockwise and then counterclockwise like a circle.
3. Complete three sets of 5 to 10 reps, alternating to the left leg; increase your reps, sets, or both when your strength permits.
4. Wait at least 1-minute in-between sets.

Note: Hold on to the back of a chair or any stable object if necessary:

———————————————

Lying Down

Muscle groups activated by the ankle circles:

◆ Legs (calves, ankles, and feet)

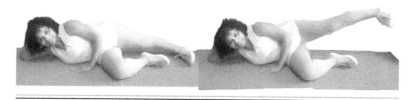

Lying down ankle Circles:

Perform Lying Down, Standing, or Seated:

To Begin:

1. Start by turning your ankle around slowly in circles to the left, then to the right.
2. Lead with your big toe.
3. Keep your movements small and focus on only your foot and ankle, not your entire leg.
4. Complete three sets of 5 to 10 circles alternating legs. Increase your reps, sets, or both when your strength permits. Wait at least 1-minute in-between sets.

FULL BODY ANATOMY

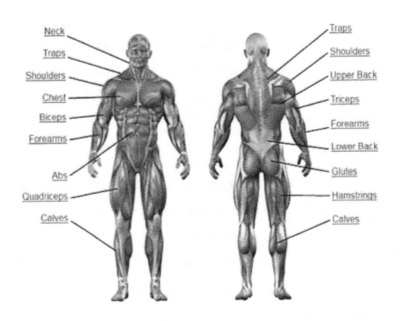

End-Book Review Page

Strength in Numbers

Now that you are armed with everything you need to know to build your strength and flexibility daily, you are in a perfect position to help me get the word out to others.

By sharing your honest opinion of this book and your experience with the exercises, you'll show new readers where they can find everything they need to improve their health and fitness.

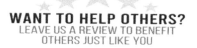

WANT TO HELP OTHERS?
LEAVE US A REVIEW TO BENEFIT
OTHERS JUST LIKE YOU

I appreciate your support – I could not do this without you.

CONCLUSION

We have come to the end of the book. We have tried to cover all the body's major muscle groups to give you a well-rounded exercise experience. Many of the exercises illustrated can be performed either seated, standing, or lying down. It's been our goal to offer exercises in different planes, not knowing the physical fitness level of the reader. If you have a physical limitation, one of the three options may work for you. We have tried to tailor each muscle group exercise with variations so that whatever your fitness level, or condition, there is an exercise to match your current condition and fitness level. As a senior citizen, I realize the need to do something with my body to challenge it through strength exercises to live a healthier life. If there is a takeaway from this book, it should be the importance of movement in your life and a commitment to stay committed to an exercise regimen in some way for the rest of your life. I am often asked, "How long should I continue these exercises," and my answer is always the same. You should continue with some form of exercise for the rest of your life if you want a chance to enjoy good health longer into your senior years. You may rest and take some time off occasionally, but resting differs from quitting. Take your rest, but never quit. Always make the commitment to continue, and by continuing, the results will make it all worth it. You will live a healthier life, and statistically, you will live longer. As one famous author once said, "You can have what you want. You just need to make up your mind". If it is a healthier body, you can have that. We need to decide to achieve it. In this case, I hope you continue strength exercises; if you do, it will be among the best decisions you will ever make.

———————————

References

stretching -exercises-for-seniors. (n.d.). Https //ioraprimarycare.com/blog/stretching-exercises-for-seniors/. Retrieved October 10, 2022, from https://https //ioraprimarycare.com/blog/stretching-exercises-for-seniors/

Sign in - Article Forge. (n.d.). https://af.articleforge.com/users/sign_in?enable_me trics=1

stretching -exercises-for-seniors. (n.d.). Https //ioraprimarycare.com/blog/stretching-exercises-for-seniors/. Retrieved October 10, 2022, from https://https //ioraprimarycare.com/blog/stretching-exercises-for-seniors/

Vanner, C. (2020, November 9). Quick & Easy Exercises Seniors Should Do Every Day. ActiveBeat - Your Daily Dose of Health Headlines. https://activebeat.com/your-health/senior/quick-easy-exercises-seniors-should-do-every-day/

9 Hip Strengthening Exercises for Seniors. (2022, April 20). Iora Primary Care. https://ioraprimarycare.com/blog/hip-strengthening-exercises-for-seniors/

Phlips Lifeline. (2021, February 9). 14 Exercises for Seniors to Improve Strength and Balance. Lifeline. https://www.lifeline.ca/en/resources/14-exercises-for-seniors-to-improve-strength-and-balance/

Balance Exercises for Seniors. (n.d.). PureGym. https://www.puregym.com/blog/5-of-the-best-balance-exercises-for-seniors/

Kerkar, P. (2018, November 21). 8 Best Neck Exercises To Prevent Neck Pain. Epainassist. https://www.epainassist.com/back-pain/upper-back-pain/8-best-neck-exercises-to-prevent-neck-pain

You Can Still Work Out Your Upper Body From a Chair. (2021, July 15). Verywell Fit. https://www.verywellfit.com/seated-upper-body-workout-1231439

Lord, E. (2022, September 7). Seated dumbbell wrist curl. WeightTraining.guide.

https://weighttraining.guide/exercises/seated-dumbbell-wrist-curl/

Bodybuilding.com. (n.d.). Seated Bent-Over Two-Arm Dumbbell Triceps Extension | Exercise Videos & Guides. https://www.bodybuilding.com/exercises/seated-bent-over-two-arm-dumbbell-triceps-extension

Burchette, J. (2022, December 28). How to Do an Overhead Triceps Extension (Video). The Beachbody Blog. https://www.beachbodyondemand.com/blog/overhead-tricep-extension

Pelvic Floor Muscle (Kegel) Exercises for Males. (2023, January 24). Memorial Sloan Kettering

Cancer Center. https://www.mskcc.org/cancer-care/patient-education/pelvic-floor-muscle-kegel-exercises-males

Patterson, A., sr. (2021, June 17). <u>10 Best Back Strengthening Exercises for Seniors</u>. Careasone. Retrieved September 9, 2022, from https://careasone.com/blog/10-best-back-strengthening-exercises-for-seniors/

<u>Build Your Biceps With Dumbbell Curls</u>. (2022, November 7). Verywell Fit. https://www.verywellfit.com/how-to-do-the-biceps-arm-curl-3498604

Malik. (2019, April 28). <u>Seated Bent-over Two-arm Dumbbell Kickback (Triceps) | Exercise Guides</u>

and Videos. Fitness Volt.

https://fitnessvolt.com/24107/seated-bent-over-two-

arm-dumbbell-kickback/

Patterson, D., Sr. (2021, June 1). Bent Over

Lateral Raise | Illustrated Exercise Guide. SPOTEBI.

Retrieved November 13, 2022, from

https://www.spotebi.com/exercise-guide/bent-over-

lateral-raise/

Elsevier – Patient Education | Sit-to-stand

exercises. (n.d.). https://elsevier.health/en-

US/preview/sit-to-stand-exercises

From Weak and Wobbly to Strong and Stable.

(n.d.). Eldergym Fitness for Seniors.

https://eldergym.com/shoulder-exercises/

Davis, N. (2019, March 8). 10 Medicine Ball Moves to Tone Every Muscle in Your Body. Healthline. Retrieved September 10, 2022, from https://www.healthline.com/health/fitness-nutrition/medicine-ball-workout

Jackson, J. (2022, May 2). Resistance band forearm exercises and workouts for muscle growth. Critical Body. https://criticalbody.com/resistance-band-forearm-exercises/

Biswas, C. (2022, November 23). 15 Best Wrist Strengthening Exercises To Avoid Pain & Injury. STYLECRAZE. https://www.stylecraze.com/articles/exercises-to-strengthen-your-wrists/

Nash, S. L. (2022, May 25). The 18 Best Abs Exercises You Can Do Standing Up. Greatist. https://greatist.com/move/abs-workout-best-abs-exercises-you-can-do-standing-up

14 Ab Exercises You Can Do While Watching Netflix in Bed. (2022, March 1). Byrdie. https://www.byrdie.com/best-at-home-ab-exercises

HASfit. (2016, November 14). 20 Min Chair Exercises Sitting Down Workout - Seated Exercise for Seniors, Elderly, & EVERYONE ELSE. YouTube. https://www.youtube.com/watch?v=azv8eJgoGLk

Stelter, G. (2017, December 19). 5 Gentle Back Pain Stretches for Seniors. Healthline.

https://www.healthline.com/health/back-pain/stretches-for-seniors

The Back Workout You Can Do At Home - - Really. (2022, February 1). Shape. https://www.shape.com/fitness/workouts/back-workout-6-moves-blast-annoying-bra-bulge

Walle, M. G. S. van de. (2022, October 27). 8 Simple Stretches to Relieve Lower Back Pain. Healthline. https://www.healthline.com/nutrition/stretches-for-lower-back-pain

McCoy, J. (2022, April 23). 15 Quad Exercises That Seriously Smoke the Tops of Your Legs. SELF. https://www.self.com/gallery/best-quad-exercises

Jones, R. C., & Turco, L. C. del. (2021, November 3). 15 Hamstring Exercises That'll Seriously Sculpt Your Legs And Booty. Women's Health. https://www.womenshealthmag.com/fitness/a19962155/hamstring-exercises/

https //www.webmd.com/pain-management/knee-pain/injury-knee-pain-16/slideshow-knee-exercises - Google Zoeken. (n.d.). https://www.google.com/search?q=https+//www.webmd.com/pain-management/knee-pain/injury-knee-pain-16/slideshow-knee-exercises

Kelly, E. (2022, February 17). Eight of the Best Hip Flexor Stretches and Exercises. Healthline. https://www.healthline.com/health/fitness-exercise/hip-flexor-exercises

Kelly, E. (2022, February 17). Eight of the Best Hip Flexor Stretches and Exercises. Healthline. https://www.healthline.com/health/fitness-exercise/hip-flexor-exercises

Made in the USA
Las Vegas, NV
27 November 2023

81617392R00203